I am 50 years old and I have Menopause

Chapter 1: Menopause; a sickness or a stage in life

The period after the second world war saw such phrases like;

"You've made some amazing progress, infant"

becoming   a repetitive motto. The statement mirrors the struggles that had preceded the post-war phase. The expression indeed says a great deal regarding the ladies of this age. One minute, you are a young girl just trying to get through her first period. Acne dysmenorrhea and pre-menstrual symptoms all over the place and you being so confused about it all. The next minute, you are in your fifties, going through irregular bleeding and experiencing perimenopausal symptoms and still as confused as you were when you first saw your period.

 Irrespective of whatever you think you know, or what you have achieved or established in this life, you realize that you know so little when menopause is concerned. At the same time, you realize how far you have come n you start to approach menopause. There used to be a time when the issues of the sexual and reproductive health of women was a hush topic. Today however, women have made some fantastic progress in opening up the conversation about surrounding these women issues, particularly, menopause. The expression "you've made some amazing progress, infant" closes with "however you have far to go." Women today may well live 40 or 50 years after menopause. This effectively puts menopause right around the middle of their lives. This leaves space for so many more things to happen for and to these women beyond the shores of menstrual decline. There is still room for so much to go right, or go wrong and it all starts with that very first symptom.

In this part, we acquaint you with menopause, its symptoms, presentation and implications. **Characterizing Menopause**

from the moment a female child is born, it is a countdown to puberty. and from that point of puberty, it is yet another countdown to menopause. The puberty period of women is loosely defined as the period a girl child gradually reaches sexual and reproductive maturity. Menopause is when the girl, now a woman, begins to achieve a decline in her reproductive prowess. These are two very important phases of life and they share numerous attributes. Some people refer to them as the two advances. These periods in a woman's life are so important because they are the hallmarks of gender and sex. Considering the sheer amount of mental and emotional strain they both place on women, it is a lucky thing that they don't last forever. These two phases in a woman's life are set off by hormones; the two of them cause physical and emotional changes (that could make a person appear insane), and the two of them close a few entryways and open new ones. Adolescence is the point at which the hormones in a girl's body originally gets the ball rolling.

 Girls generally remember this period differently in their lives. Even though the girls didn't know it at the time, the reproductive hormones in their bodies spiked, resulting in physical changes such as appearance of the breasts, broadening of hips, thinning of the voice, and growth of hair on pubic areas. Many girls experience changes in emotions due to hormone and hormonal fluctuations in the brain. Over a couple of years though, their hormones would slowly regulate into a more balanced formulary and an agreeable level. The periods, which had been irregular earlier would finally settle, into a predictable cycle, and their emotional equilibrium pretty much re-established.

The body remains like this for years (all things being equal.) The fertility of girls in this stage is at an all-time high. In fact, researchers have found that this period between the age of 15 and 25 are the best times to have healthy births. by the time the woman reaches age 35-40 though, the reproductive prowess reduces significantly, mostly because of a slow but steady decline in the concentration and regularity of the hormones. At some point, the reproductive hormones drop and reduce so much that it starts to affect the basic reproductive functionality of the woman's body. Some of the expected changes that come with menopause are

1. Night sweats
2. Irregular menstrual cycle
3. Anovulation
4. Hot flushes
5. Heavy period bleeds
6. Irritability
7. Vaginal dryness (and as a result, painful intercourse)
8. Susceptibility to yeast infection
9. A complete stop of menstruation
10. Headaches etc…

Once Again, the hormones settle into a new norm of lower production. With this comes an eventual complete disappearance of periods after some time of inconsistency.

Getting The Wording Right

Have you at any point seen how you don't give close consideration to bearings or where you're going when you're the traveller in a vehicle? You just begin to stress over each leave number and stoplight when you're the one in the driver's seat. Menopause is that way. You catch wind of menopause and menopausal manifestations. Yet, you rarely give a lot of consideration to the specifics until it's your turn. At the point when you do slide into the driver's seat and begin focusing, you might become baffled by the wrong wording related to the entire menopause experience. Besides the leaflets you get from the specialist's office, most books, magazines, and articles that deal with menopause like a phase that begins with hot glimmers and continues for the remainder of your life. This book hopes to do better by you by breaking it all down into simple language while also being intentional about the use of proper words for phenomenon surrounding the topic. Here is a brief description of each of the identified keywords relating to the conversation we are about to have.

Menopause

Menopause implies the finish of the menstrual cycle. During the years on the way to menopause (called perimenopause), your periods might be unpredictable to the point that you're never sure which period will be the final remaining one. Yet, you're not authoritatively menopausal until you haven't had a period for a year.

Perimenopause

The term perimenopause alludes to the time frame that ushers in the end of the menstrual cycle when estrogen creation is easing back down. Many indications that people generally name as menopausal (hot blazes, disposition swings, restlessness, etc.) occur during the perimenopausal years.

It is important to differentiate the perimenopausal period from menopause itself because a non-differentiation of the two phenomena can result in serious mistakes and consequences.

We likewise use the term "perimenopause" because we need to note the physiological and enthusiastic changes women experience preceding the finish of your periods and recognize them from the progressions that occur after your body has acclimated to bring down degrees of estrogen.

Post menopause

The time after your last period is called post-menopause. However, this word has never honestly gotten on. The term "post menopause" is frequently used to refer to the actual occasion and the years after menopause. At the point when we talk about menopausal ladies in this book, we're discussing ladies who have quit having periods — regardless of whether they're 55 or 75. The years paving the way to and following menopause mark a major transformation in a lady's life. As you clear your path through this time of your life, you'll realize two major things.

1. That you have finished a chapter in your life that was crucial to your identity as a woman.
2. That you are about to begin yet another delicate chapter, and that the possibilities are endless.

The changes in your body and your life will most likely not come suddenly. They usually come in slow phases, revealing the many changes that will occur over time. Here's a short description of the stages related to menopause.

Moving toward the change: Perimenopause

Perimenopause is the stage during which your hormones begin to change gears. A few months during which your hormones work at the levels they've worked at for as far back as 30 years or somewhere in the vicinity; other months, your maturing ovaries don't deliver estrogen when they ought to. Your cerebrum reacts to this absence of estrogen creation by sending a signal to attempt to get those ovaries kicked off. When they receive the signs, your maturing ovaries overcompensate but are unable to deliver estrogen in the identical amounts that they used to. Your period is late because your ovaries created less estrogen during the initial segment of your normal cycle or because you may never have ovulated, making the entire process abnormal and surprising — you may experience abnormally heavy or light flows due to this irregularity. During this period of perimenopause, you may have your period. However, you are likely to experience side effects that people who are approaching menopause do. On the off chance that you go to the specialist at this stage and ask,

"What's happening to me? Could this be menopause?"

The specialist will most likely go directly to the "Could this be menopause?" part of your inquiry depending on your age and medical history. You will not be considered menopausal if you still have periods, even if they are far apart and irregular. There have been many cases of misdiagnosis in relation to Peri menopausal and menopausal health challenges. Numerous specialists miss the initial segment of the investigation — the "What's happening to me?" part. This is the main problem you need to make quick work of — the reason for your unusual and disturbing health experiences.

Discharging no more: Menopause

Menopause is often deemed to be only associated with monthly bleeding that requires a sanitary towel. Many specialists believe that menopause becomes official when a woman has missed her period for a year. Ladies can become menopausal roughly between age 35 and 50. The definition may appear to be straightforward from the outset, yet there are a couple of circumstances that may leave you scratching your head.

If you have been using hormonal treatments that for example require you take estrogen for a few days and progestin during the last couple of days of your cycle. You may experience a semblance of a period (the progestin makes your body shed the coating of the uterus even if you have not naturally ovulated). The question then becomes whether or not you are menopausal? Now, another scenario would be one in which you have been deferring your last period by taking adequate measurements of estrogen to free yourself of perimenopausal symptoms. your body, may at this stage act almost completely normally and you may have yourself and your doctor wondering whether you are menopausal. If you are, at what stage exactly did it happen and which symptoms are strictly perimenopausal and which ones are associated with other things? Here's another interesting one: If you've had a hysterectomy (careful expulsion of the uterus), you're viewed as "precisely menopausal." But, if you had your uterus eliminated, but kept your ovaries, no doubt about it menopausal because your ovaries produce estrogen. By taking your blood and testing it for your hormone levels will enable your doctor to determine and reveal whether your hormones are formally at menopausal levels.

These precarious circumstances bring up critical questions as to what exactly defines menopause. the one thing that remains common to all menopause related questions is that of the hormones. The principal worry here is what's going on with your hormone levels, particularly estrogen. Hormonal changes can trigger numerous physical and psychological medical problems.

When you arrive at menopause, your hormone production levels are so low that your periods stop. Your ovaries produce some estrogen and testosterone; however, instead of delivering hormones in cycles (which is why you have periods and why you're fertile for reproduction for around four or five days every month), your body presently creates consistent, low quantities of hormones. The kind of estrogen your ovaries produce additionally changes from a functioning sort to a relatively idle version which is really unable to do much in the way of reproduction stimulation.

Moving beyond menopause: Post menopause

Post menopause is the time of your life that begins after menopause (a year after your last period) and closes when you die. This is the point at which your body is living on extraordinarily diminished degrees of estrogen, testosterone, and progesterone. In this book, we will only discuss both the suspension of your period and your life after that as a menopausal woman.

Expecting Menopause

When will you get menopausal? The circumstance differs from one lady to another. Foreseeing it is highly unlikely to be precise science. You can't even make guesses based on the time difference between when you started to have periods and when your peers and girls in our age group experienced the same. many factors come into play here such as genetics, diet, lifestyle etc… in the end, menopause happens on its own timetable.

we have drawn up some calculated guesses that will answer the question of "when am i likely to experience menopause?'. Most ladies become perimenopausal at some point between the ages of 35 and 50. You'll most likely know it when you arrive because you'll presumably have a portion of the indications (look at the Cheat Sheet at the front of this book and Chapter 4) and add some unpredictable periods. it is particularly typical to experience menopause itself at some point in their 50s. There are of course exceptions to this rule as established by lifestyle, genetics and pre-existing medical conditions. these factors make room for unusual occurrences that lead to a couple of known uncommon kinds of menopause. Below is a list of such unusual menopausal experiences.

Untimely menopause

This basically happens when ladies go through menopause in their 30s, usually before the age of 40. This is considered abnormally early. It could happen as a result of genetics or some other medical condition.

Clinical menopause

Alludes to menopause prompted by chemotherapy, radiation, anorexia, or different medical conditions. This sort of menopause is now and again reversible. However, your periods may require a month, or even a much longer time to return.

Careful menopause

Alludes to menopause induced by a medical procedure. Evacuation of the two ovaries, for instance, induces a quick, non-reversible menopause. Since your ovaries produce a wide range of sex specific hormones **(estrogen, progesterone, and testosterone),** any surgery that amputates the ovaries is going to bring about a very stressful period for the woman. She will go straight into significant menopausal presentations like hot flushes and the end of the menstrual period is instantaneous.

Chapter 2: Midlife Transition

As the baby boomers born between 1946 and 1965 grow older, a more significant number of women are making the transition to menopause than in past decades. Many of us in this generation want to understand our bodies to make informed decisions. Our large numbers have stimulated interest in menopause-related research and treatments. Some view us as a market for often unnecessary and sometimes even harmful tests, services, and interventions. Despite this increased focus on menopause, many of us still feel uncertain about what to expect because it is becoming increasingly clear that most of the stakeholders I need for the money and not necessarily because they care about women and their experiences. It definitely doesn't help that recent lifestyle changes amongst women have created a completely new and increasingly diverse experience and reality when it comes to menopause. From increased stress levels due to workplace competition with men, to diet, lifestyle changes, medications and even environmental exposures.

Today, we find ourselves wondering, "What's normal?" Does everyone else feel this way?" or even "Does *anyone* else feel this way?" We may ask, "Why can't our periods just stop without all these other physical changes and emotional roller coasters? What is going on in our bodies?"

This chapter describes the changes most women experience as they make the transition to life after menopause. It also explains how our bodies produce various hormones throughout our lifetimes—and the effects these hormones may have on us. The last section of the chapter provides an overview of problems—such as sleep disruption, depression, and memory and sexual concerns— that some women experience during the menopause transition.

There is a wide range of typical experiences of the menopausal transition. No two women will have the same experiences. Most research suggests that menopause-related development occurs gradually over a decade or more. Most women notice changes— such as hot flashes—but these last for no more than about five years. Every woman who survives to midlife will experience menopause naturally if she has not already experienced it because of surgery, medical treatment, or other causes.

The typical transition to natural menopause is a gradual process, with increasing irregularity of menstrual periods and eventually, a final menstrual period occurring at about age fifty-one, the average for U.S. women. Smokers have their last period one to two years earlier than non-smokers, on average. (This difference may be due to decreased blood flow to the ovaries in smokers or the toxicity of tobacco to the ovaries.) The changes in our bodies that precede menopause may begin as long as a decade or more before our last menstrual period. Researchers are just starting to understand some of these changes, as most women's studies during the menopausal transition have not included women in their late thirties and early forties. Some of us experience natural early menopause, with our final menstrual period occurring before we are forty years old. Some women experience induced menopause due to chemotherapy or radiation therapy or removal of both ovaries (bilateral oophorectomy), which often accompanies the removal of the uterus (hysterectomy).

When a gathering of ladies talks about their encounters of pubescence, menstrual cycles, and pregnancy, the narratives are everywhere. A few ladies don't see changes in their bodies; others perceive the second ovulation or origination. A few ladies have horrendous issues with premenstrual disorder (PMS); others experience difficulty-free cycles all through their whole lives. Ladies' encounters shift with perimenopause and menopause similarly; however, much they differ with these different changes. In this part, we cover what you may gain insight as you start the transition into perimenopause.

Beginning

Most ladies' ovaries start experiencing a change at some point between the ages of 35 and 50. If your periods end before you arrive at 40, you have experienced what's known as untimely menopause. Perimenopause is once called a climacteric period, which implies that it's a significant period. Recollect that your ovaries don't simply close down one day; the progress is filled with ups and downs that may create a rollercoaster of physical and psychological symptoms and side effects. Perimenopause is a period of significant physiological change — when egg creation alongside the support of estrogen and progesterone starts easing back down.

Recognizing indications

We give Chapter 4 only to the manifestations ladies may experience during perimenopause. A few different parts clarify the connection between your hormones and these symptoms. Not up to 50% of all ladies experience irritating side effects like hot Flushes, heart palpitations, rest intrusion, and emotional episodes during the transitional period before menopause. Most ladies who have these symptoms experience the side effects of hormonal fluctuations and imbalance. In contrast, Different ladies perceive that they're perimenopausal because their periods, which used to be pretty much predictable, become grossly unpredictable. Their periods might be late, or even completely refuse to show. Do my experience ridiculously light menstrual period, or it may come as heavy as a flood. Lamentably, while a doctor can make calculated guesses based on your symptoms there are no tests that specifically test for perimenopausal condition

Bringing In The Experts

Suppose you're in your late 40s or 50s, and you're encountering the symptoms recorded on the Cheat Sheet and in Chapter 3. There is a significantly higher chance that you're perimenopausal. You should however still consult your physician just to be sure that this is the situation. There are many intersections between the symptoms of perimenopause and thyroid issues, cardiovascular infection, clinical depression, and other genuine medical problems. Your clinical specialist can properly diagnose you and also help you manage the bothersome indications of perimenopause and forestall real medical issues that are more predominant after menopause.

Owning it as far as possible

Since you never truly know when perimenopause begins, precisely characterizing a time is troublesome. A few ladies experience symptoms for a very long time before their periods stop. The truth of the matter is that most of the symptoms you find out about are brought about by the fluctuating hormone degrees of perimenopause instead of the maintained, low degrees of hormones you experience during menopause. You're authoritatively menopausal one year after your last period. From that point forward, numerous individuals utilize the term post menopause to stamp the remainder of your life (however, in this book, we simply continue to use the word "menopause").

Advancing Longevity

In the not-so-distant past, 50 was probably as old as possible to hope to get. Today, many of us will live ways into our 70s, 80s, and 90s. The fact that most ladies quit being reproductive in their 40s doesn't imply that some ladies are not, at this point, Able to carry healthy and term pregnancies after 40. With the entire reproduction issue far removed, ladies have additional time and freedom to make new commitments to life on earth (or in space).

Experts have identified some important keys to long and cheerful premenopausal and postmenopausal life. They found that the ability to accept the new reality is a big factor for most women. Another key is taking adequate care of yourself and the rates you're managed. Standard exams can address clinical issues as they emerge and help forestall others. Eat suitable food varieties (and parts), get some activity, and carry on with life to its fullest. Everybody agrees that a tangible course of action is to attempt to diminish problematic perimenopausal side effects, forestall sickness, and advance a long and sound life. It's likewise the most un-hazardous technique for managing perimenopause and menopause. Responding to this call requires self-evaluation and a touch of the-end. Moving to a reliable way of life includes prevention of unfortunate propensities, getting, in any event, a half-hour of high-impact workout five times each week, and keeping a sound, adjusted eating regimen that incorporates, at any rate, five servings of plant-based food every week.

THE TRANSITION YEARS

To communicate more clearly about menopause, a team of researchers and health care providers recently proposed a set of terms and definitions to de- scribe its stages.

The **reproductive stage** is the time in a woman's life when she starts menstruating until the menopausal transition begins.

Perimenopause is a term for the menopausal transition, which rese archers divide into early and late stages.

Menopause is defined by a woman's last menstrual period. Because women's periods can be sporadic just before menopause, studies usually require that a woman has not had a period of one year to qualify as having experienced menopause.

Postmenopause begins after menopause (the last period). Like perimenopause, it can be divided into early and late stages. Early post-menopause includes the first five years after the final period when the hormone changes that started before menopause have stabilized. The late post-menopause extends throughout the remainder of the lifespan and occurs when ovarian hormones have reached a new, steady lower state.

Menstrual calendars

In addition to having irregular periods during the menopausal transition, women also frequently experience spotting (scant bloody discharge) before, after, and between menstrual bleeding episodes. Some of us also have longer and heavier bleeding episodes (menorrhagia or flooding). Some have shorter periods and minor bleeding. Some women have a rapid change in bleeding patterns and some experience irregular periods over more than five years.

Stages of reproductive ageing

The late stage of the menopausal transition occurs when a woman skips her usual period so that her cycle becomes double the length that is typical for her. The menopausal transition may start in our early to mid-forties. However, there has not been sufficient research with younger women to be specific. Estimates from studies over the past two decades suggest that women experience irregular cycles for about five to six years before menopause.

Women participating in the Seattle Midlife Women's Health Study have kept daily menstrual calendars shown here for fifteen years. These women's experiences suggest that the early menopausal transition stage begins at an average age of forty-six years old and lasts for an average of nearly three years. The late menopausal transition stage begins at about age forty-nine and lasts for about two years. Women in the Seattle study reached menopause at an average age of nearly fifty-two. The earliest menopause recorded at almost forty-four years old and the latest at fifty-nine.

Changing hormones

The start of the menopausal change is heralded by irregular periods in ladies who have had regular cycles already. The progressions in a lady's periods are a sign that changes are happening in her ovaries. The advancements in our ovaries are organized by a perplexing arrangement of signs from hormones in the brain, pituitary organ, and ovaries themselves. Hormones help control the basic and complex functionality of the body. Reproductive hormones are responsible for the development of follicles (or egg sacs) in the ovaries. Follicles contain eggs (ova) that develop until the time has come to deliver one of them from the ovary. This happens each cycle, making Fertilization and implantation possible. Apart from carrying the ova, the follicles produce hormones, including estrogen; the hormone that is responsible for attributes of our bodies related to being female, for example, the development of breasts and the hair covering the vagina. The ovaries likewise make androgens, hormones commonly connected with the help of "male" fundamental qualities like hair growth and muscle development and improvement.

How would I know when I'm menopausal?

The most dependable approach to gauge where you are in the menopause lane is to monitor your periods on a schedule like the one on page 44 for a couple of months. Every day you can stamp on the program whether you have had to die (B) or to spot (S). You can distinguish when you are in the early menopausal change stage when the length of your periods contrasts by possibly more than seven days starting with one cycle then onto the next. However, you have not yet begun skipping periods. A few of us have unpredictable processes for our entire lives. As far as we might be concerned, utilizing a menstrual schedule doesn't help pinpoint where we are in the menopausal change. Monitoring our cycles might be valuable for different reasons, for example, pregnancy arranging, fertility treatment, or following exceptionally hefty periods before we counsel our medical services supplier for help. Following a couple of long stretches of following your period on a feminine schedule, follow these means:

1. Looking at the schedule for your last periods, tally the length of your cycle by starting with the principal day you have denoted a B for dying. At that point, check every one of the days with a B set apart, in addition to the days that have either an S (spotting) or a clear until the beginning of the following draining days (stamped B). Rehash this for, in any event, two cycles.

2. Take away the number of days for the second cycle from the number of days for the principal process. (It doesn't make any difference if you get a positive or negative number).

3. If the difference in the number of days between cycle one and cycle two is at least seven, you might be in the beginning phase of menopausal progress. (Note: This won't function admirably on the off chance that you have had irregular cycles for the more significant part of your life.)

4. If there are sixty days or more between the beginning of menstruation in one cycle and the following, or if the days are about to double your typical cycle length, you might be in the late

menopausal progress stage. When you arrive at this stage, the odds are that you are inside two years of your last fertile period. This is bound to be the situation if you have had an example that resembles the early menopausal progress prior.

Follicle-stimulating hormone

During the reproductive stage, follicle-stimulating hormone (FSH), which comes from the pituitary gland in the brain, signals the ovaries at the start of every cycle to produce more estrogen by causing ovarian follicles to develop. FSH works something like a thermostat on a furnace, with estrogen being like the heat produced.

When FSH rises, the amount of estrogen the ovaries produce increases. When estrogen levels reach a high-enough set point, FSH decreases.

Myth or reality?

• After menopause, ladies experience the ill effects of estrogen inadequacy; we either have estrogen levels that are excessively low or have no estrogen at all.

Ladies don't quit producing estrogen altogether after menopause, rather, our estrogen levels become lower. When ovulation and monthly cycles stop, we make estrone, a less dynamic kind of estrogen, by changing androgen over to estrogen in fatty tissue. Estrone keeps on furnishing our body with a wellspring of estrogen after menopause.

• There seems to be a correlation between the experiences of mothers and daughters.

It isn't clear if this claim is valid or bogus as there is little proof from investigations of moms and girls to determine hereditary qualities in menopause. There is proof that ladies whose moms had early menopause are bound to have early menopause. It is however questionable whether girls or ladies who had menopause-related health issues around the time of menopause are bound to have a close encounter.

As we approach our last Menstrual periods, the quantities of follicles in our ovaries are a lot more than at the height of our reproductive prowess. This prompts a quick drop in the quantities of follicles remaining accessible for the future turn of events such as ovulation, and pregnancy. The immediate improvement of more hairs can bring about the creation of higher degrees of estradiol, the most dynamic type of estrogen, for specific months or years. The quick improvement of follicles is connected to rising degrees of FSH. FSH levels usually increment progressively until a little while before the last menstrual period, when they increment quickly.

Inhibin

Inhibins are proteins in the ovaries that help control the ovulation process through their effects on FSH. Inhibin A and B keep FSH levels low during the reproductive years. Inhibin levels drop in the years before menopause at the same time that FSH levels rise. The drop in inhibin B levels reflects the diminishing number of follicles left for future development in the ovary. As the number of follicles available to develop decreases below the level necessary for ovulation, ovulation stops.

Progesterone

Progesterone is a hormone
produced by the ovaries in the last two weeks of the   menstrual

cycle after ovulation occurs. It helps prepare the lining of the uterus (endometrium) so that a fertilized egg can implant. When ovulation stops, progesterone is no longer produced. Thus, as the menopause transition is completed, there is a shift in the balance of hormones to have much less estradiol and no other progesterone from the ovaries.

Androgens

Androgens are often thought of as male hormones, but women produce androgens in their ovaries and the adrenal cortex. The adrenal cortex is the outer layer of cells of the adrenal gland, which is located next to our kidneys. The adrenal gland secretes several hormones that our bodies can make into androgen. Some of these are called dehydroepiandrosterone sulphate (DHEAS), dehydroepiandrosterone (DHEA), and androstenedione. Our ovaries also produce the hormone testosterone. Testosterone levels do not change dramatically during the transition to menopause, although they do decrease with ageing. DHEAS levels also decline with age in both women and men.

DHEAS can be metabolized to either a potent androgen   or   to estrogen, providing an adrenal source of androgen and estrogen for

women after menopause. Androgens are responsible for male-appearing sexual characteristics, such as hair growth and distribution on the body, muscle growth, and deepening of the voice.

Sex hormone-binding globulin

Sex hormones restricting globulin (SHBG) are related to hormones in the blood. They connect to receptors in the cells of different tissues, accordingly delivering the hormones all through the body where these receptors are available. SHBG diminishes by around 50% from when a lady is in her mid-twenties until her late forties, with the most significant drop two years before menopause. This drop-in SHBG permits hormones like estradiol or testosterone to be more effective and concentrated in the body. Diminished SHBG levels happen simultaneously as the drop in estradiol levels women experience with the menopausal change. The free androgen record, determined as the proportion of testosterone to SHBG, increases by 80% during this period, with the maximal change happening two years before the last menstrual period.

When SHBG drops, more androgen opens up at about the very time that estradiol drops. This can bring about the impacts of androgen turning out to be all the more noticeable. A few of us have expanded hair development on our upper lip or face. We may Develop a more masculine fat appropriation (fat on the midsection rather than on the thighs and bottom). Skin break-out can re-emerge. Many women find these progressions in our bodies alarming. Yet, others may not experience them at all or may not be disturbed by them.

Estrone

As the amount of estradiol produced by the ovaries decreases with approach to menopause, the adrenal gland provides an essential source of another type of estrogen called estrone. Women have this estrogen before and after menopause by converting androstenedione (a type of androgen) to estrone. Estrone is a much weaker estrogen than estradiol.

Signs of the menopausal transition

Some of the symptoms associated with the onset of menopause include hot blazes and night sweats; depression; sleep disturbance; sexual performance concerns; changes in perception (thinking and judgment); vaginal dryness; urinary incontinence; and head throbs and agony. A couple of these become substantially more common as ladies progress through the change to menopause. Hot blazes, night sweats, vaginal dryness, and rest interruption are the most common, particularly as ladies start the late menopausal change stage set apart by skipping periods.

How long these issues persevere during post-menopause is questionable because most investigations have not followed ladies for more than a few years after their last menstrual period.

Hot flashes

Nearly four in ten women are bothered by hot flashes during the late menopausal transition stage and post-menopause. According to one large study, about 26 percent of women have severe hot flashes; according to another study, 15 percent of women experience hot flashes on more than fifteen days per month, and 9 percent experience them every day.

Your invitation to share my story came just as I experienced the fourth hot flash of the day. I was, as usual, dripping with sweat and wiping my brow under my breasts, the back of my neck, and my hands so I could continue working at the keyboard. Fortunately, I work at home, so I can strip down when necessary. Occasionally, though, I do media work. It can be pretty inconvenient to sweat away from the makeup that someone has just carefully applied! Anyway, this has been going on for more than two years now, but I can say some days are worse than others. It's worst of all at night, and in the first year, I sometimes was awakened every hour with its intensity. I get hot enough to steam up my glasses—something that evokes unfailing sympathy from my husband, who keeps saying he can't imagine how I can cope with it. I tell him I'm not alone, and there are millions of baby boomer women out there going through the same thing.

Chapter 3: Symptoms of menopause

From an unusually bad temper, mood swings to difficulty resting, heart palpitations, and a certainty that someone keeps sneaking the indoor regulator up when you're not looking. Sound familiar?

Assuming this is the case, you're very likely at the beginning of menopause. Each human body is unique, and when it comes to menopause, nothing is necessarily unexpected. Be that as it may, the experience of menopause uncovers exactly how extraordinary we genuinely are. A few ladies breeze through the change, encountering not very many actual distresses or bombshells. Others have a hailstorm of medical problems for many years. Luckily for most ladies, the indications frequently pass as they move into menopause and past. In this part, we give a prologue to the perimenopausal and menopausal symptoms that they may experience.

The indications we examine in this section are, for the most part, manifestations of perimenopause or menopause. Yet, they're not limited as symptoms to only for perimenopause or menopause. Other ailments — or even typical varieties — cause these symptoms also. Some of these symptoms can appear on their own or in relation to other medical conditions, so it is important to get checked out if you experience any of them. Your primary care physician will help you preclude any more real purposes.

Kicking Things Off with Perimenopausal Symptoms

We have mentioned some perimenopausal and menopausal symptoms in various parts of this book. But in this section, we are going to concentrate on the many presentations that have been credited to the unexpected drops of estrogen during perimenopause. The symptoms of menopause or perimenopause will not always show up in all women. In fact, many ladies in the United States report encountering no perimenopausal indications at all. For ladies who experience side effects, the manifestations can go in seriousness, from being mildly irritating to serious medical conditions that make them doubt and question their will to be alive

Getting physical

On the off chance that you do have actual manifestations as you enter and go through perimenopause and menopause, you may discover them challenging to overlook. They're, indeed, extraordinary. Individuals frequently compare arriving at menopause and hitting pubescence, however moving toward maturity didn't involve hot flashes, balding, sleeping disorder, or heart palpitations. A considerable lot of the actual indications are the aftereffect of a series of occasions that are gotten underway when estradiol (the dynamic type of estrogen — the "great" stuff) levels

Unexpectedly drop — a run-of-the-mill event during perimenopause. The drop causes a chain response inside your body, which we depict in the "Noteworthy the science behind the indications" sidebar later in this section. The connection between estrogen and serotonin assumes a part in the significant number of psychological side effects. However, it additionally contributes to a portion of the actual indications — like rest interruptions. Serotonin is a compound that assists the body with controlling rest and temperaments. Even though every one of the subtleties isn't in, estrogen plays some part in the creation and upkeep of serotonin.

Turning up the warmth

Hot flushes are particularly common in menopause — 85% of ladies have them at any rate once or twice as they enter perimenopause, and 10 to 15 percent of ladies report having them regularly enough or seriously enough to look for clinical treatment. At the point when you have a hot flush, you unexpectedly feel hot and exceptionally flushed — particularly in your face and chest area. Expanded sweat — anything from a clammy upper lip to enough perspiration to leave your clothes or bed sheets awkwardly wet — as a rule, happens as a result of this warmth. Also, some of the time, Confusion, heart palpitations, and a stifling inclination can go before or go with hot glimmers.

An abrupt drop in estrogen levels triggers a hot flush. This drop-in estrogen tells the brain that something is seriously off-base, so your cerebrum sends a large dose of adrenaline (norepinephrine). This is the hormone that triggers the fight or flight reaction in people, so your body moves into the prepared mode, which gets your pulse up and your heart beating and causes the veins in your brain, neck, and chest to expand. This disturbance causes that boiling feeling. Until 1970, specialists didn't recognize hot flushes as a genuine physical phenomenon; they ascribed the sensation to a psycho-coherent issue. Indeed, however, the impact of hot flushes is tangible and quantifiable — ask any individual who's consistently slept close to a lady when she experiences hot flushes. Her skin temperature may go up as much as six degrees, as though she had a fever. Thankfully, this side effect is just brief, ordinarily lasting close to 10 minutes or somewhere in the vicinity. Hot flushes aren't terminal. However, the first few experiences of it may cause panic unless you've been warned to expect them.

Perspiring and night sweats

Night sweats are hot flushes that happen around evening time. A similar estrogen drop that triggers hot glimmers during the day starts night sweats. Night sweats can likewise be caused by infections, thyroid issues, or different kinds of ailment, so if this is the only perimenopausal symptoms you experience, check with your PCP.

Losing your resting time

With every one of the peculiar manifestations continuing during the day, getting a decent night's rest so you can awaken feeling rested doesn't should not be too much to ask, but it very well may be; however, the absence of rest during this period can be a genuine issue. Hot glimmers in the night regularly bring about disturbed rest. You awaken, regularly sweating (and a few times reviling), with clammy bedsheets and skin that may wind up being bothersome as you cool off and all that sweat dries, and struggle returning to rest. If your rest gets disturbed often in this way, you can develop a significant rest deficit, which could cause crabbiness, tension, and emotional episodes.

Serotonin is a hormone that is found all through your body, particularly in your brain. A synapse is a substance that sends messages starting with one nerve cell then onto the next. There's still a great deal we don't understand about serotonin and its capacities. However, it can act to influence our muscles, nerves, and mindsets. A fast drop in estrogen additionally controls your serotonin levels. Serotonin directs disposition and sleep medications. (Medications, for example, Prozac and Zoloft, work on the rule that serotonin guideline is vital to easing emotional episodes, touchiness, etc.) Estrogen makes serotonin more accessible by drawing out its activity. When estrogen drops, it influences your serotonin levels, which adds to rest and sleep disturbances.

If somehow, you manage to get a good night's sleep in the middle of your perimenopausal cycles, you ought to inform your PCP as this might be an indication of abnormal cells creating in the covering of your uterus that ought not to be disregarded.

Getting to the core of the palpitation issue

The unexpected drops in estrogen that are so regular during perimenopause cause responses everywhere on your body (see the "Noteworthy the science behind the indications" sidebar later in this part), including heart palpitations. The drop in estrogen causes your body's natural painkillers and mood stabilizers (endorphins) to drop. Your body deciphers this situation as an inconvenience, so it sends an explosion of adrenaline (norepinephrine, the fight or flight Hormones). Your body then reacts as you had suddenly encountered a large mountain bear. The problem is, you didn't see the wild bear, and you could be left wondering why your heart is beating so fast at that moment even though you were just seated to eat a sumptuous dinner.

The way to deal with menopause can be different for various feminine changes. Yet, you need to realize that you can't put all abnormalities on perimenopause. Discuss with your medical care supplier about the accompanying abnormalities and any remaining indications before essentially writing them off to perimenopause:

Anticipating feminine inconsistencies

Sporadic periods are fundamental in perimenopausal ladies because fluctuating hormone levels can intrude on the ovulation cycle. A few months you ovulate; a few months you don't. If you don't ovulate, you don't have a favorable situation to produce enough progesterone to have a period.

Heavy bleeding during perimenopause usually is brought about by an "eggless" cycle. This happens when you make estrogen during the initial part of your process, yet you don't ovulate for reasons unknown. Subsequently, you don't produce progesterone. You build up an unusually thick uterine lining, which you shed during your period.

Random, unexpected blood shows could be a cause for embarrassment in many women. One perimenopause will make managing your periods simpler because it is nearing an end. The reverse is the case and however long you have periods, they're likely to appear on poorly timed occasions this can make you really happy to be Rid of them.

Uncovering the science behind the indications

As you may have suspected, the indications of menopause are primarily attached to plunging hormone levels. You may feel these side effects more during perimenopause than menopause itself because your hormone levels change more during perimenopause. At times they climb to genuinely typical levels, and afterward, they come slamming down. The variance is the trigger for a ton of the manifestations. In menopause, hormone levels are reliably lower than during your conceptive years, so they don't spring up and drop down so often. However, manifestations can, in any case, happen. Here's a bit-by-bit guide of what befalls your body when your estradiol (the dynamic type of estrogen) levels drop:

1. Your ovaries produce lower estradiol levels, which causes a drop in the measure of estradiol arriving at the cerebrum.

2. Less estradiol in the cerebrum causes a lessening in your endorphin levels. Endorphins are your body's characteristic painkillers and mood controllers and regulators. (In case you're a sprinter, you're presumably acquainted with the impacts of endorphins — they cause the "sprinter's high.")

3. Lower levels of endorphins in your mind cause it to feel that something is off-base. Hence, it conveys an explosion of adrenaline, particularly norepinephrine (the hormone that triggers the fight or flight reaction).

4. The explosion of norepinephrine makes your body kick into prepared-for-anything mode by expanding your pulse (which causes those palpitations and pauses), raising your circulatory strain, and widening your veins. Expanding veins cause hot flushes and perspiration. In case you're sleeping, you may awaken out of nowhere. You may likewise encounter the runs or get a sensation of tension and butterflies in your stomach.

Taking care of the migraines

For ladies who experience headache cerebral pains preceding or during the initial few days of their periods, we have some terrible news — you may have more migraines during perimenopause. During the initial few days of your period, cerebral pains imply that you're touchy to low estrogen levels, which are typically around then. When estrogen levels drop rapidly, which occurs during perimenopause, the drop may trigger another of those cerebral pains. Similarly, as your estrogen level has gotten capricious, so may your migraines. Again, as you're complimenting yourself for being without a migraine in June, July may bring on a whopper.

Confronting the fibroid titbits

Fibroids are essentially chunk of uterine muscle tissue. Almost 33% of ladies have fibroids when they're 50. Fibroids will, in general, get bigger and more disturbing as you approach menopause. Yet, they ordinarily don't keep on increasing in size after menopause. You genuinely don't have to do anything about fibroids except if they cause side effects like torment, pressure, or bleeding. Similarly, as with different indications, talk with your

PCP if you're having any issues, you feel might be identified with fibroids.

Playing head games

The psychological/passionate indications related to perimenopause can be disappointing. Numerous ladies don't connect their new touchiness or depression with perimenopause. For the most part, symptoms we list Notwithstanding, these indications seriously burden or, in any case, trouble numerous ladies during perimenopause.

If this portrayal reflects your circumstance, there's no compelling reason to stay there enduring peacefully. Make sure to inform your clinical expert about these psychological and enthusiastic indications. They might be more firmly identified with distinctive hormonal characteristics than with mental issues. In any case, your medical care proficient can guarantee that you get the legitimate therapy to ease your symptoms.

Sitting on the emotional episodes

Emotional episodes are regular among perimenopausal ladies. However, remember that emotional attacks are likewise frequent before your period (part of premenstrual symptoms) and after pregnancy. Although clinical specialists don't know about every one of the details, low levels of estrogen are related to lower levels of serotonin, which can prompt emotional episodes, notwithstanding crabbiness,

Agonizing over uneasiness

Nervousness is another typical side effect perimenopausal ladies face. Similarly, as with temperament and mood swings, tension is by all accounts attached to low degrees of estrogen. The lower levels of endorphins and serotonin related to low estrogen levels may trigger uneasiness. Another hypothesis is that low degrees of estrogen, serotonin, and endorphins leave you more powerless against the emotional stressors in your environment. As indicated by this hypothesis, lower estrogen, serotonin, and endorphin levels don't trigger uneasiness; they essentially limit your capacity to manage upsetting circumstances.

Addressing fractiousness

The very hormonal movements that cause mood swings and tension (see the past "Sitting on the emotional episodes" and "Stressing over nervousness" areas) cause crabbiness. Similarly, as with these different manifestations, checked fractiousness is a transitory condition that appears to blow over after you're formally menopausal (if that you can endure yourself for that long).

Reviewing memory glitches

Memory issues during perimenopause sneak up on you. You fail to remember your companion's name one day; you leave your keys someplace in the supermarket another day. Soon, you begin recollecting how often you were unable to recall something. We're not discussing dementia or Alzheimer's illness here; we're talking about carelessness and an absence of core interest that happens due to hormonal imbalances in the brain. This classification covers moderately minor memory glitches: You fail to remember where you're going with an idea in mid-sentence, or you get to the store and fail to remember what you need to purchase. Thank heavens for sticky notes and essential food item records.

Estrogen appears to work with correspondence among neurons (nerve cells) in the cerebrum. Quite a bit of memory involves the cerebrum sending data starting with one memory stockpiling focus then onto the next. Since estrogen keeps up associations and develops new ones, changing and imbalances in estrogen levels can hinder correspondence between memory caching territories. Memory issues appear to be a short-term issue; most ladies appear to lose the memory slips after menopause. Signs from later phases of the Women's Health Initiative appear to be that for ladies. More seasoned just, hormone treatment is related with an increment in the danger for dementia and, in general, psychological working. Since this is something contrary to what analysts in this enormous, 15-year study anticipated they'd find, follow-up investigations of the connection between hormone treatment and a decrease in psychological working are ongoing. There's no authoritative word yet on the impacts of hormone therapy in more youthful ladies on dementia, psychological working, or memory. Even though the Women's Health Initiative Study revealed a genuinely massive expansion in the danger of dementia among ladies somewhere in the range of 65 and 79 who were utilizing either mix (estrogen in addition to progestin) hormone treatment, the general danger of Alzheimer's in the United States is still significantly and comparatively low.

Thoroughly considering a fog

Fluffy reasoning is normal and expected when you're denied rest or your hormones are in transition. At the point when we say smooth reasoning, we mean the inclination that you're only not with it today — like you're strolling through a haze or you can't focus on the thing you're doing. Fluffy reasoning can be the aftereffect of sleep and rest disturbance (which is incredibly basic during perimenopause). Fluctuating hormone levels likewise cause fluffy deduction (as you may have experienced during pregnancy or at specific focuses in your menstrual cycle). Fluffy thinking is not a permanent change and will likely resolve as you go into full swing menopause. For the most part, it clears up when your hormones settle down, and your rest designs relax during menopause. Encountering little mind flatulates every so often doesn't imply that you're on the elusive slant to untimely mental feebleness — this will pass.

Visiting the Menopausal Symptoms

Every one of the manifestations we portray as perimenopausal has for quite some time been credited to menopause. However, after you're menopausal (without a feminine period for a year), things start to settle down a piece. Hot blazes die down, and your temperaments settle. Your body and mind appear to become accustomed to certain parts of lower estrogen creation. A few ladies may keep on encountering menopausal symptoms for quite a long time after their periods end. The manifestations experienced after menopause may even be a smidgen more awkward actually. On the off chance that this is you, don't simply endure it as you don't have to — work with your physician to help you track down a hormonal or non-hormonal treatment to keep you agreeable.

To keep away from monotony, we utilize the term menopause in this section (and most others) to allude to the time frame that fuses both menopause and post menopause.

Sorting out the actual realities

After you formally arrive at menopause (following 12 Whole months without a Menstrual period), you produce lower estrogen levels without the unexpected spikes and drops an average of perimenopause. Your hormones quiet down — route down. As time passes by, these significant stretches of low estrogen levels bring about some actual changes. In this segment, we talk about what these conditions feel like. We expound on the science behind these conditions and lighten the manifestations in different parts of this book. A portion of the symptoms is the consequence of lower levels of estrogen, straightforward as can be. We call these essential manifestations. A part of these crucial indications can create additional repulsiveness, which we call optional side effects.

Taking a gander at the essential side effects

The critical side effects incorporate

Vaginal dryness

The clinical foundation alludes to this condition as vaginal decay. Since estrogen keeps vaginal tissues saturated and moist, consistent low estrogen levels can bring about the drying and contraction of vaginal tissue. Somewhere in the range of 20 and 45 percent of ladies in the United States experience vaginal dryness. They frequently notice it when intercourse gets excruciating because of an absence of lubrication.

Vulvar uneasiness

Tingling, consumption, and dryness of the vulva aren't unusual amongst menopausal ladies. In any case, note that numerous conditions and illnesses that influence the vulva have nothing to do with estrogen, so have your primary care physician look at any vulvar changes.

Urinary incontinence

This condition is substantially more pervasive in ladies during perimenopause and menopause than during their previous conceptive years. The tissues of your urinary system become drier and slenderer, and the muscles lose their tone as estrogen levels lessen. You know you're experiencing urinary incontinence if you struggle to hold it when you giggle, exercise, or sniffle. Your urinary parcel, particularly your urethra, depends on estrogen to keep up its structure and muscle tone. The urethra struggles to fix off the progression of pee following quite a while of decreased estrogen levels.

Urinary recurrence

Like incontinence, urinary recurrence results from maintained, low degrees of estrogen that characterize menopause. Urinary recurrence implies that you need to pee constantly. You may leave the restroom and rapidly feel like you need to go once more. This condition can be exceptionally baffling during the day — and surprisingly more disappointing around evening time. Urinary recurrence can likewise cause interference with rest, which justifiably transforms into peevishness.

Cerebral pains

Ladies who experience their first headache during perimenopause regularly track down that the headaches disappear after menopause. Headaches are very common during the perimenopausal stages. Women who experience headaches as a pre-menstrual symptom or pregnancy symptoms are also very likely to experience it in perimenopause.

Skin changes

Lower estrogen levels cause your skin to lose immovability and flexibility. Estrogen doesn't, in a real sense, forestall drooping or wrinkles. However, estrogen keeps your skin flexible and assists your skin with holding liquid, so it stays "rounded out" instead of getting free and sagging.

Hair changes

Your hair gets more slender and more fragile with menopause. However, a few ladies report that their hair feels as delicate and comfy as cotton quite a while into menopause. Estrogen appears to advance your body's regular creams, so with lower levels of the stuff moving through your body, your hair endures a shot and turns out to be more fragile and wirier. You additionally make some more complicated memories keeping a perm lasting. However, a few ladies likewise note that their hair has more body than it used to and find that they at this point don't have to cleanse consistently to keep their now moderately drier hair looking great.

Weight changes

Your weight movements to the focal point of your body — around your midsection. Rather than the beautiful hourglass shape you once had, you take on a more significant amount of an apple-molded appearance because of moving hormone levels. However, you may acquire a touch of weight, you likely can't straightforwardly put that on hormonal changes. Your body just turns out to be less lenient about wholesome uneven characters and helpless eating, drinking, and exercise propensities.

Prompting the optional conditions

It's not finished at this point. At least one of the essential manifestations can trigger significantly more un-enjoyableness. Here you go:

Difficult intercourse

Vaginal dryness and changes within the vagina can prompt distress or torment during intercourse. As low degrees of estrogen may cause your uterovaginal tissues (tissues of the vagina and urinary plot) to become slender and the supporting muscle to lose its tone, your organs typically shift position apiece.

Sleep and rest disturbances

Hot flushes, urinary recurrence, uneasiness, and an assortment of other menopausal side effects can intrude on rest during the evening. You awaken tired and feel exhausted for the day because your body can't enter the profound phases of rest around evening time that cause you to feel tough and fiery.

Exhaustion

On the off chance that you reliably don't get a decent tranquil night's rest or you experience sleep deprivation, you may get exhausted. In any case, weariness can likewise be the consequence of low testosterone levels.

Finding that it's more than shallow

The psychological/energized parts of menopause are even more a hodgepodge. A few manifestations experienced during menopause typically decline or disappear totally; others are a smidgen harder to manage.

Uneasiness

The uneasiness regular during perimenopause is frequently brought about by the fast drop in estrogen, which starts a chain response (see the "Uncovering the science behind the indications" sidebar prior in this part). After menopause, unexplained tension regularly fades away, and you get back to your typical self.

Gloom and depression

Ladies who have had hysterectomies are bound to encounter menopause-related melancholy than are ladies who go through characteristic menopause. Scientists don't yet comprehend why this is the situation. Yet, almost certainly, physical, mental, and social factors all have an influence. Likewise, ladies who have been on estrogen and unexpectedly quit taking it, instead of going through a weaning cycle, additionally have more issues with depression. Estrogen aids the creation of serotonin (a substance that manages dispositions), so lower estrogen levels can mean lower levels of serotonin.

Lower sex drive

Diminished sex drive is an issue for some menopausal ladies. However, fortunately, 70% of ladies remain explicitly active during their perimenopausal and menopausal years. Lower moxie can be followed by an awkward hormonal nature and might result from testosterone levels being shallow.

Memory slips and fluffy reasoning

Even though memory slips and fluffy reasoning are regular during perimenopause, most ladies notice their concentration and memory recover to business as usual after menopause. Age can cause mental weakness further down the road, yet you can't put everything on menopause! However, keep in mind If you are yet utilizing hormone treatment now, talk with your PCP about whether the reasons you proceeded with hormone use to this point are yet legitimate.

Chapter 4: Nutrients and Menopause—Vitamins, Minerals, and Special Nutrients

Sufficient intake of vitamins, minerals, and particular nutrients is an integral part of the Six-Step Healthy Menopause Program. This chapter tells you all about them and explains the many functions they perform in terms of menopause. Phytoestrogens and essential fatty acids are mainly featured. Nutrients are workhorses, required components of hundreds of hormone reactions continuously taking place within body cells and supporting life. When your body sends signals that it is hungry, nutrients are what it asks for, not just calories. Browse through the following information on vitamins, minerals, and particular nutrients to understand just how important each one is for female health. And for an overview, take a look at the section at the end of this chapter that lists various menopausal symptoms and the most effective nutrients for treating them.

Food Sources of Nutrients Versus Supplements

Suppose you are barely troubled by menopause and eat a balanced diet. In that case, you may be consuming sufficient amounts of nutrients through the everyday foods you eat. However, most individuals would benefit from also taking vitamin and mineral supplements. You can't always trust food to supply you with what it's supposed to contain. If produce is grown on land depleted of minerals, the mineral content of the food will also be lower. Transporting, processing, and storing foods also destroys the nutritional value of many food products. And suppose you are troubled by menopausal symptoms, which can be a sign of nutrient deficiencies. In that case, you will most likely need to take supplements in therapeutic dosages. You could never eat enough food to consume the higher quantities of nutrients required to treat specific symptoms. You'll find a list of suggested nutrients and the amounts to take later in this chapter.

Vitamins

Without vitamins, your body would not be able to function. Having sufficient levels of vitamins and enzymes speeds the making or breaking of hormone bonds that join molecules together. These reactions drive cellular activity and make the production of energy possible. If you reach menopause low on vitamins, deficiency symptoms such as fatigue and irritability can show up— problems blamed on menopause that simply may be the result of poor eating habits. The information in this chapter tells you what foods are exceptionally high in the various vitamins. If you rarely eat many of these foods, start adding them to your grocery list. A warning about cooking such foods: Vitamins have more delicate and unstable chemistry than minerals. Since vitamins can be readily destroyed in cooking, each of the following sections concludes with tips on cooking foods to preserve these fragile nutrients.

Vitamin A and Beta-Carotene

Vitamin A, a fat-soluble vitamin, is found in meats and other animal foods. In contrast, the *carotenoids,* a family of water-soluble vitamins with vitamin A activity, are supplied by plant foods. One type of carotenoid, beta-carotene, is well known. Still, there are over 400 different carotenoids, each important for health in their way. Carotenoids are red and yellow pigments—the coloring agents that give red peppers, carrots, and golden acorn squash their hue. All green vegetables also contain beta-carotene, but the stain can't be seen because the green chlorophyll masks it.

Benefits

•Vitamin A is essential for skin growth and repair, thereby helping to maintain moist outer skin and inner vaginal tissue.

•Vitamin A helps slow physical changes that begin to show up post-menopause.

•Beginning at midlife, a woman's night vision may begin to decline, making such activities as night driving much more difficult. Night vision depends upon having adequate stores of vitamin A. Through a series of hormone reactions, the vitamin A you consume becomes part of the photoreceptor cells in the eye that make it possible for you to differentiate between light and dark.

•With age, hair may lack luster, which is also a sign of vitamin A deficiency.

•Vitamin A stimulates the immune system, and beta-carotene in particular acts as an antioxidant, destroying free radicals that can lead to cancer.

Best food sources of vitamin a

Vegetables: sweet potatoes, carrots, butternut squash, spinach Fruit: cantaloupe, mango, apricot Meats: beef and calf's liver (preferably organic) Dairy: butter (preferably organic) Miscellaneous: eggs

Cooking tips

•To preserve fat-soluble vitamin A in meats, avoid cooking them at very high temperatures. Frying meats damages their vitamin A by oxidizing it. Sauté meats and roast at lower temperatures for a longer time instead.

•To maximize your intake of the carotenes, cook carotene-containing vegetables so that the cell walls break down and release the vitamins, which are then easier to absorb. Steam or bake carrots and yellow squash, excellent sources of this vitamin, and better yet, serve these vegetables puréed or mashed. This method of preparation turns familiar foods into new and exciting dishes.

B-Complex Vitamins

There are 11 B-complex vitamins. The most well-known are thiamin (B1), riboflavin (B2), niacin (B3), pantothenic a cid (B5), vitamin B6 (pyridoxine), B12 (cobalamin), and folic acid. The remaining four are choline, inositol, biotin, and para-aminobenzoic acid (PABA). These latter four are present in the liver, eggs, unprocessed whole grains, and molasses. The complete complex of B vitamins works together to nourish the nervous system and stabilize brain chemistry. These vitamins are essential for converting food into energy and help maintain healthy skin and hair. Stress uses up B vitamins, which can become depleted by such body changes as menopause.

Thiamine, B1

Benefits

•Thiamine supports the health of the nervous system. A deficiency of B1 can result in irritability.

•Thiamine helps keep the mind sharp. A lack of vitamin B1 is associated with an inability to concentrate and memory loss, which can occur

during menopause. best food sources of thiamine whole   grains: rye, rice, wheat, millet, buckwheat, bulgur Beans: pinto, black, garbanzo, soy, black-eyed peas Vegetables: potatoes, peas, Jerusalem artichokes, corn, okra Fruit: watermelon, avocado Nuts: Brazil nuts, pine nuts, pistachios Seeds: sunflower seeds Meats: pork, liver, quail Fish: lobster, trout, oysters

Cooking tips

Thiamine is the second least stable vitamin after vitamin C. Because it is water-soluble, chopped and minced vegetables can lose up to 70% of this vitamin in the cooking liquid—a good reason to save the juice for soups. Cook potatoes in their jackets. Thiamine is stable in acidic-based foods but not in alkaline-based foods, so baking powder in baked goods can cut by half the amount of thiamine present in flour. The thiamine in meats, fish, and poultry is best preserved by roasting, broiling, and braising and is reduced by stewing and frying.

Riboflavin, B2

BENEFITS

•Strengthens adrenal function, thereby supporting hormone balance and lessening susceptibility to menopausal symptoms

•Generally slows the ageing process by helping maintain good vision, healthy

hair and nails, and youthful skin, including vaginal tissue

•Helps sustain energy by increasing the ability of the cells to use oxygen

BEST FOOD SOURCES OF RIBOFLAVIN

Whole grains: wild rice, millet, wheat

Fish: clams, salmon, mackerel, trout, herring Vegetables: yams, mushrooms, winter squash Fruit: avocado Beans: pinto, black Meat: liver (preferably organic), dark-meat chicken Nuts: almonds, hazelnuts, chestnuts, cashews Seeds: pumpkin Dairy: milk, yoghurt

COOKING TIPS

•Light is the greatest destroyer of riboflavin, but this is not usually a problem since milk products and bread are generally stored in the dark. Nuts and seeds should also be kept away from light.

•Riboflavin is diminished when food is chopped and cooked, especially when the food is cooked in a lot of liquid since riboflavin is water-soluble. Steam or bake instead. Enjoy some riboflavin-rich foods, raw, and whole.

Niacin, B3

BENEFITS

Helps stabilize blood sugar, which, when fluctuating dramatically, can trigger a range of menopausal symptoms

•Supports mental clarity and memory, since niacin plays a role in brain metabolism

•Increases energy by improving circulation

•Sustains sexual function by benefiting vaginal tissue and stimulating the formation of mucus in response to sexual activity

•Lowers cholesterol

BEST FOOD SOURCES OF NIACIN

Meat: liver, beef, chicken, turkey Fish: tuna, salmon, halibut, oysters, shrimp, sardines Vegetables: mushrooms, potatoes, asparagus, broccoli, summer squash Fruit: peaches, cantaloupe Nuts: peanuts Whole grains: whole wheat, corn tortillas (To make corn tortillas, Mexicans soak their maize in lime water overnight to free the niacin in the grain from its inactive bound form.)

COOKING TIPS

•Niacin is very stable. Cooking a food containing niacin makes the vitamin easier to absorb.

•When you cook meat, water-soluble niacin accumulates in the meat juices. By making a sauce from the juices, you can add the niacin to the dish you are preparing.

Pantothenic Acid, B5

BENEFITS

•Essential for optimal adrenal function and necessary for hormonal health post menopause

•Helps in the management of stress by increasing the production of the adrenal hormone cortisone, thereby reducing the frequency and severity of menopausal symptoms

•Necessary for proper brain function

•Aids in the prevention of premature ageing and wrinkling of the skin

BEST FOOD SOURCES OF PANTOTHENIC ACID

Meat: beef liver (preferably organic), chicken Fish: bluefish, abalone, trout, salmon, cod Fruit: avocado, pomegranate

•Raw foods are the best source. Pantothenic acid is easily destroyed if heat is coupled with ingredients that are especially acidic or alkaline, such as vinegar or baking soda.

•The low temperatures used in deep freezing can destroy pantothenic acid. However, pantothenic acid's presence in such a wide variety of foods may compensate for its fragility.

Choosing the Best Form of Key Nutrients

If you shop for supplements, you'll find that vitamin C comes in capsules but is also available as a powder. Natural vitamin E is on the market, but stores also sell synthetic vitamin E. Minerals are not sold in their pure form. Instead, bottles list calcium as calcium carbonate or calcium citrate. This section explains which forms of these nutrients are the most beneficial.

Vitamin C

Vitamin C is an acid—ascorbic acid—, and in high doses, it can cause gastric dis- comfort. A less acidic alternative is sold in powder form under the trade name Ester-C ascorbate, which is more easily absorbed than regular vitamin C and is better utilized by body tissues. Another bonus of Ester-C ascorbate is that it does not erode tooth enamel. Plain ascorbic acid can cause severe damage to teeth, especially if you take chewable vitamin C, which comes in direct contact with your teeth. For insurance, whenever you take any form of vitamin C, be sure to rinse your mouth afterward with filtered water. Vitamin C remains in your system for only about 4 hours before it is excreted in the urine. For this reason, take vitamin C in divided doses throughout the day. The first sign of overdosing is diarrhoea.

Vitamin E

Natural vitamin E is made from vegetable oils and consists of one particular molecule called D-alpha-tocopherol. Some natural vitamin E supplements also contain mixed tocopherols. These are beta, gamma, and delta tocopherols, which have less vitamin E activity in the body but are also beneficial. Synthetic vitamin E is made from petroleum or turpentine and is a mixture of eight molecular configurations, seven of which are human-made and do not occur naturally. Synthetic vitamin E is referred to as dl-alpha-tocopherol. Natural vitamin E appears to be more beneficial than synthetic vitamin E. It is better absorbed into organs and tissues. In addition, some researchers question whether synthetic vitamin E ties up receptor sites, preventing any natural vitamin E present from acting. To be sure your vitamin E is 100% natural, look for the following on the label: independently assayed to guarantee 100% potency, 100% natural source. As vitamin E is an oil-soluble vitamin, there is the possibility of overdosing and toxicity. Signs of toxicity include nausea, diarrhoea, intestinal gas, headache, heart palpitations, and fainting. Dosages recommended for menopause are many times greater than the RDA. However, even in these more significant quantities, signs of toxicity are rare. To gauge how much vitamin E you can tolerate while taking a sufficient amount to decrease menopausal symptoms, increase your intake slowly. Begin with 400 international units a day, continue this for two weeks and, then add another 400 in- global companies every two weeks until you notice symptoms such as hot flashes subsiding. Stop increasing the dosage when it reaches 1600 international units a day. If you decide to cut back, reduce your intake by 400 global companies is in 2-week intervals.

Calcium

Calcium carbonate provides the most concentrated form of calcium. It is adequately absorbed if taken with meals. Look for factory-made kinds rather than natural calcium carbonate in the form of bone meal, oyster shell, or dolomite, which may contain lead.

Other forms of calcium supplements include calcium phosphate, calcium lactate, calcium gluconate, calcium maleate, and, most importantly, calcium citrate. This form of calcium is much better absorbed than other forms and is widely available. However, one drawback of calcium citrate is that it can increase the absorption of aluminium, leading to kidney disease and is linked to Alzheimer's disease. If you take calcium in this form, make sure the deodorant you are using does not contain aluminium. In addition, avoid eating food cooked in aluminium pots and pans. Note that some restaurants such as diners use this cheaper type of cookware. If you want to check how easily your calcium supplement dissolves, indicating how easily it may be absorbed, place a calcium tablet in 6 ounces of white vinegar or apple cider vinegar. Set this aside for 30 minutes, stirring occasionally. A top-quality calcium tablet should dissolve within this period. For maximum absorption, take calcium in divided doses, two to three times a day. With each amount, also take some vitamin C, which increases absorption of this critical mineral. Some people find that calcium makes them feel relaxed and even tired, so you may want to take it before bedtime.

Special Nutrients

Besides the familiar vitamins and minerals just described, nature provides other vital nutrients to assist your passage through menopause. These nutrients include bioflavonoids, compounds similar to vitamins, phytoestrogens, substances that behave like hormones within the body, and essential fatty acids, a group of fats that promote good health. Many common foods contain these nutrients, but a diet of fast foods only provides a meager amount. To ensure an adequate intake, you need to turn to the simple fare of whole foods described in Chapter 5. For now, let's take a look at these nutrients, what they consist of, and how they behave within your body tissues.

Bioflavonoids

Bioflavonoids originally called P vitamins, are not vitamins. They are a group of water-soluble compounds that include citrin, hesperidin, quercetin, rutin, flavones, and flavonols. A combination of these is often included in vitamin supplements for women. In foods, bioflavonoids are accompanied by vitamin C, a variety that al- lows for better absorption of the bioflavonoids. Citrus is a rich source of these vitamins, with lemons containing the entire complex. The central fluffy white stem within citrus fruits includes the highest concentration of bioflavonoids. The hormone formula of specific bioflavonoids resembles that of estradiol, the primary form of estrogen. These bioflavonoids display hormone activity similar to this hormone.

BENEFITS

Bioflavonoids help control hot flashes. They are also used to lessen the psychological symptoms of menopause, including anxiety, irritability, and mood swings. Bioflavonoids strengthen capillary walls, thereby curbing heavy menstrual bleeding that can occur during perimenopause. This action also helps reduce the likelihood of varicose veins, spider veins, haemorrhages, and black-and-blue marks. Rutin is particularly effective in preventing varicose veins. Bioflavonoids help slow the ageing process in other ways too. They work in conjunction with vitamin C to prevent ruptures in connective tissue, keeping skin firm and healthy. And the bioflavonoid quercetin helps prevent cataracts.

GOOD FOOD SOURCES OF BIOFLAVONOIDS

Fruit: black currants; grapes; plums; cherries; apricots; blackberries; papaya; cantaloupe; the pith, membranes, and central white core of citrus including oranges, lemons, limes, and grapefruit Vegetables: green peppers, tomatoes, broccoli Whole grains: buckwheat Miscellaneous: rose hips

COOKING TIPS

Bioflavonoids are very stable compounds, minimally affected by heat, air, and light. They are present even in canned fruits and vegetables.

Phytoestrogens: Hormones from the Plant Kingdom

Many common foods contain compounds that have the capability of behaving like hormones within the human body. These have been given the popular name of phytoestrogens. Such compounds first drew the attention of scientists in the 1940s when it was observed that sheep in many parts of Australia were becoming infertile. The ewes stopped ovulating. The problem was eventually traced to the red clover on which the sheep were grazing. The animals were taking in about 1 gram a day, a considerable amount. Such extremely high doses can stop ovulation. Birth control pills function the same way. By the 1970s, attention turned to the effects of estrogens in the human diet. Scientists began measuring the phytohormone content of dozens of vegetables, fruits, grains, seeds, and flavorings routinely used in cooking that shows some degree of estrogenic activity. These days the research focus is on the effect of all these phytoestrogen-rich foods on symptoms of menopause. In addition, their potential ability to lower the risk of heart disease and breast cancer is being ad- dressed.

WHY PHYTOESTROGENS ARE IMPORTANT FOR F EMALE HEALTH

Phytoestrogens function as modulators and have a balancing effect on hormone levels. They play a dual role, mimicking the functions of estrogen when supply is low and dampening it when too much is available. Phytoestrogens bind to estrogen receptor sites, such as those found in breast tissue. This blocks the body's own more potent form of estrogen from attaching. Because of the lower potency of phytoestrogens, this substitution, in effect, reduces estrogenic activity. But when the body produces only a tiny amount of estrogen, plant estrogens contribute to this supply. However, as Bruce Milliman, N.D., associate professor adjunct faculty at Bastyr University in Seattle, states, "The impact of phytoestrogens on the system goes way beyond their activity at binding sites. They can also mimic estrogen as well as impeding the breakdown of estrogen." And, he continues, "In addition, the functions of phytoestrogens may also depend on the ratio of various types of estrogens within a woman's body. And diet can be an important part of the equation. So, the questions and answers are very complicated."

SUBTLE POTENCY BUT POWERFUL EFFECTS

Although estrogenic substances in foods have been shown to affect hormone status, phytoestrogens have potencies that are far, far weaker when compared with the effectiveness of estradiol, the primary form of estrogen made by the ovaries.

Phytoestrogens have only 1/400 to 1/100,000 the potency of estradiol. However, specific eating methods can provide a significant number of photos- estrogenic ingredients, making a difference. In a landmark study, women living in rural Japan who ate a diet high in estrogenic soy foods were found to have levels of phytoestrogens in their urine in quantities 100 to 1000 times greater than that of women United States. Japanese women have a much lower incidence of hot flashes: fewer than 20% of them than 80% of North American women experience this symptom. The Japanese language doesn't even in- include a word for "hot flash." Various studies have also shown that women who eat a vegetarian diet may have phytoestrogen levels 100 times greater than women eating a typical North American diet.

NUTRIENTS FOR THE SYMPTOMS OF MENOPAUSE

Hot flashes: niacin, pantothenic acid, vitamin C, vitamin E, chromium, magnesium, potassium, selenium, bioflavonoids, phytoestrogens, essential fatty acids

Fatigue: niacin, pantothenic acid, vitamin B12, folic acid, vitamin C, vitamin E, calcium, iodine, iron, magnesium, manganese, potassium

Mood swings: riboflavin, vitamin B5, chromium, bioflavonoids, ph ytoestrogens

Anxiety and irritability: thiamine, riboflavin, pantothenic acid, folic acid, vitamin C, vitamin D, vitamin E, calcium, copper, magnesium, manganese, phosphorus, potassium, bioflavonoids, essential fatty acids

Depression: vitamin B6, magnesium

Poor memory: thiamin, niacin, pantothenic acid, vitamin B12, folic acid, iodine, essential fatty acids

Vaginal thinning and loss of elasticity: vitamin A, riboflavin, niaci n, vitamin B6, vitamin C, vitamin E, copper, selenium, essential fatty acids

Vaginal lubrication: niacin, vitamin C, vitamin E, selenium

Libido: zinc

Fluid retention: vitamin B6

Irregular cycles: phytoestrogens

Heavy menstrual flow: bioflavonoids, vitamin C

Chapter 5: Natural or holistic medicines, do they help eradicate menopause?

When it comes to treating perimenopausal/menopausal symptoms, can—or should—you bypass prescription medications and instead find practical natural approaches? The answer depends on the severity of your symptoms, as well as your risk factors. If your symptoms are not especially severe, you may want to try natural approaches to see if you get any relief and get symptoms under better control to not interfere with your overall quality of life. Suppose you have issues in your medical history that should make you think twice about prescription hormones (for example, a higher risk of breast cancer). In that case, the overriding question is this: are natural methods effective for perimenopausal/menopausal symptoms? The evidence is mixed. But in practice, whether due to each woman's physiology or the skills of the practitioner,

some women do find relief from symptoms using complementary, herbal, and other alternatives. So even though we don't have conclusive evidence proving the effectiveness of some of these approaches, that does not mean you should rule them out.

Natural Supplements

One piece of advice about supplements that I think is important to keep in mind comes from holistic hormone expert Uzzi Reiss, MD. According to Dr. Reiss, we should always try supplements one at a time and give them a few weeks. That way, we can see if the supplements are working or rare, causing any side effects. Ob-gyn and menopause expert Jan Shifren, MD, hasn't seen any studies that show that natural approaches are effective for menopausal symptoms. However, she says that women indeed can try them. Though they're not FDA-approved or monitored at the end of the day, most natural approaches are probably safer than hormones or antidepressants like Paxil or Effexor. They may be no more effective than a placebo, but they are likely safer than the things I can prescribe.

I have no concerns about women trying these products, as long as I've informed them of the data. Typically, if a woman wants to try natural approaches, I say, "Why not give it a try?" I see them three months later, and if it wasn't practical, they could go to prescription therapy. As many as half of all American women seek alternative or complementary treatments for menopausal symptoms. Still, reviews of more than seventy different trials and studies have found little to no improvements using herbs, soy, mind-body techniques, magnets, electrical nerve stimulation, homeopathy, or naturopathy. The key, however, is that the trials of alternatives are usually relatively small. They do not operate in the same way that herbal and natural treatments are given to women by holistic or naturopathic physicians and practitioners, which may be the real key to success. But for researchers to "prove" something is effective enough to recommend, they need more extensive studies and more data. At the same time, the studies usually don't prove that the therapies don't work at all. It's clear, then, that some—but not all—women experience benefits. Still, you may need to employ a trial-and-error process to see if natural options are suitable for you.

MACA

While not well known,
Maca (Lepidium meyenii) is my favorite natural remedy for perimenopausal/menopausal symptoms in thyroid patients. Since the late 1980s, Viana Muller, PhD, an anthropologist, and expert in South American medicinal herbs has been making rain forest herb collecting and study trips to the Amazon River basin and the high Andes of Peru. Since that time, Dr. Muller has single-handedly championed American interest in maca, a vegetable grown in South America. Maca is a cruciferous root from the same botanical family as the turnip and broccoli. It grows at 12,500 to 14,500 feet above sea level in the high Andean plateaus of central Peru and is the most heightened growing food plant globally. It is be- lived to be one of the earliest domesticated food plants of Peru and the potato. For centuries, maca has been used by the native people of Peru as a highly nutritional food and a remedy for hormone issues like fertility, sex drive, premenstrual syndrome (PMS), and menopausal symptoms. It is rich in essential minerals, especially selenium, calcium, magnesium, and iron, and includes fatty acids, such as linolenic, palmitic, and oleic acids, and polysaccharides. Maca is an adaptogen, which means it does not increase or decrease hormone levels but instead helps the hormonal system adapt and balance itself.

According to Dr. Muller, native medicine practitioners and herbalists specifically recommend Royal Maca to

•Reduce or eliminate menopausal symptoms, such as hot flashes, vaginal dryness, and hormone-related depression, as an alternative to prescription hormone therapy

•Provide nutritional support for the endocrine system, including the adrenals, the thyroid, and the ovaries (also the testes)

•Regulate and normalize menstrual cycles Promote healthy fertility in both women and men

•Promote healthy libido and erectile function

•Support a healthy immune system without overstimulating the immune system or endangering people with autoimmune disease

•Increase energy, stamina, and endurance

The alkaloids in the maca root stimulate the hypothalamus and pituitary to produce more precursor hormones, impacting all of the endocrine glands—the pineal, adrenals, ovaries, testes, pancreas, and thyroid gland. So maca appears to be stimulating the body to produce its hormones more adequately rather than supplying hormones from an outside source. Maca also seems to have an apoptogenic effect on the immune system by stimulating the immune system. Research has shown that maca works in an entirely different way than plant hormones/Phyto estrogenic herbs/isoflavones like soy, black cohosh, and red clover. Instead, its action relies on plant sterols, which act as hormone triggers to help the body itself produce a higher level of hormones appropriate to the age and gender of the person taking it. Royal Maca also reportedly helps with thyroid function for people with Hashimoto's disease and hypothyroidism.

Now that you've been introduced to some of the prevailing attitudes toward menopause, as well as the symptoms of menopause and their origins, you are ready to begin shaping your passage through the change. The following chapters give you many tools, ranging from natural therapies to hormone replacement therapy. You'll find out about traditional remedies gathered over centuries as well as current research on menopause.

The Healthy Menopause Program takes you through this wealth of information in six easy steps. If you follow this plan, you can look forward to:

•Having solutions at your fingertips for lessening and even preventing menopause symptoms

•Being better able to manage stress and feel more relaxed

•Lowering your risk of degenerative diseases such as osteoporosis and heart disease

•Enjoying a healthy and empowering attitude toward menopause

•Having a sense of vitality and well-being

 But where do you begin? How do you pick and choose among all the information and tailor a plan of action to your own individual needs? Begin by keeping a record of how you feel. Start a menopause journal.

Your Menopause Journal

You need to develop a way of keeping a record of your menopausal symptoms that works for you. If you are always on the run, carrying a small notebook in your purse may be the only way you can be sure to write down when symptoms occur. Use a page for each day. You can accumulate helpful information this way, especially if you also write down what you've been eating or if you have had difficulty sleeping—factors that can trigger symptoms. However, thumbing through pages makes it difficult to have an overview of how you've been feeling or to decipher possible reasons why.

For this reason, even if you begin with just a notebook, you will probably soon decide to keep your notes in a calendar format. Choose a page size and configuration that suits the amount of information you plan to write down. Stationery and office-supply stores sell month-at-a-glance and week-at-a-glance calendars. Keep this calendar where you are likely to remember to write in it; for instance, it is a frequently used desk drawer at work or on a nightstand next to your bed. Using a calendar as a menopause diary allows you to easily see changes in symptoms and the patterns in which they occur. A month-at-a-glance calendar is an ideal format for tracking the regularity of the menstrual cycle during perimenopause when timing begins to become erratic. Using a calendar can also help you spot a sequence of events that ultimately trigger a symptom. What you write down can help you identify associations, leading you to write down events that you might have otherwise overlooked. For instance, you may have noticed a link between hot flashes, anxiety, and being caught in commuter traffic. Then your journal may need to include traffic data. Your own story will begin to show up in your notes as the weeks pass—a sign that you're doing a great job journaling! You may even want to work with a daily calendar divided into hours for more detailed record keeping. This format allows you to jot down what you eat when you devour it, the hour of the day you usually feel tired, and other daily habits and experiences.

Be a Sleuth

Noticing an association between symptoms and activities and events can give you clues about treating menopausal problems. For instance, let's say you note that

you routinely have breakfast at 8:00 A.M., lunch at noon, and dinner at 6:00 P.M., and you regularly write that your anxiety increases around 11:30 A.M. and between 4 and 5 P.M. each day. Such detailed journaling can give you an essential piece of information—that your concern is brought on by a lack of fuel reaching your brain, a well-known phenomenon because you haven't eaten for several hours. And now you have a solution—having a nutritious snack between meals. As you use your journal, it can become an increasingly valuable tool for managing your menopause. No one but you can gather such important information.

Charting Symptoms

If you don't particularly like writing in a diary, you can use a more straightforward format for keeping menopause records. Chart your symptoms or whatever data you want to follow. Then all you'll need to do is make a check in a box. The number of inspections will quickly give you a picture of whatever information you are recording. Set up your chart on a piece of graph paper. Across the top of the page, write the days of the week. Then, to record the frequency of symptoms, write a list of symptoms down the left-hand side of the page. This format is shown on the following page. Then take a ruler and draw lines down the page and across so that a box refers to symptoms for each day. Use the graph paper lines as your guide. When a sign occurs, make a check-in that box. Three hot flashes on Tuesday results in three statements in the Tuesday hot-flash box.

Along with this chart, you might also make a second, with days of the week across the top and an informal list of symptom triggers listed down the left-hand margin. You can use the two charts together to look for an association between symptoms and behavior for any given day of the week. A sample chart follows on page 40.

Working with the Six-Step Healthy Menopause Program

Journaling can work hand-in-hand with the six-step program for menopause. Refer back and forth between this text and your journal to figure out what changes you need to make in the way you live and what treatments you may need. The Six-Step Healthy Menopause Program gives you six powerful ways of ensuring your health as a woman. Here's a quick overview of each approach.

Step 1: Nutrients and Menopause

A wide range of vitamins and minerals plays a vital role in supporting female health. Some are particularly important for menopause. For instance, vitamin E is considered a prime menopausal nutrient, as it nourishes the reproductive system. Many other vitamins and major and trace minerals are also essential. In Step 1, you will learn about the foods that are excellent sources of certain nutrients and determine the benefits of taking nutrient supplements to make up for certain deficiencies.

Phytoestrogens are a particular category of nutrients that have been studied extensively in recent years. Menopausal symptoms can be brought on by hormone imbalances, which can be corrected with phytoestrogens. Bioflavonoids and boron, two relatively unfamiliar nutrients, also bolster female health. These compounds are subtle but powerful tools for maintaining health as you pass through menopause.

Step 2: Diet and Menopause

Good health at menopause begins with eating quality foods. Step 2 tells you all about the many naturals, unprocessed, and whole, unrefined foods women need. These foods are especially rich in nutrients that support hormonal balance and nourish various body systems. There may be some surprises for you on the list of recommended foods. New research shows that butter is better for you than margarine, and certain essential oils are required to eat! Fruits, vegetables, legumes, nuts, and seeds are high on the list, and fish is another best bet. Healthy meals are made with savory, sweet, spicy ingredients full of color and taste appeal. Foods to avoid are also covered. These are the energy and health depleters— white sugar, white flour, colas, coffee, and overly processed and fast foods of all sorts. A woman subsisting on such fare during the years leading up to menopause may enter this transition deficient in specific vitamins and minerals. This can translate into annoying menopausal symptoms and poor health later in life. Step 2 turns you into a health-wise consumer of nature's best foods.

Step 3: Herbs and Menopause

A close cousin to eating well for menopause is using herbs to treat symptoms and reverse them. Some herbs such as black cohosh and doing Quai help balance hormones. Others like chamomile are ideal for their calming effects. The range of plant substances used medicinally to treat menopause has evolved over centuries, as women have experimented with one herb and then another. In addition, many herbs have recently been put to the test in scientific studies. Today, their properties and actions are well known. If you are looking for a safe and reliable way of treating menopausal symptoms, Step 3 is an excellent place to start.

Step 4: Exercise and Menopause

This step of the Six-Step Healthy Menopause Program is not optional! You cannot expect to have good health and not move your body. Step 4 introduces you to the types of pleasurable physical exercise that have been proven to reduce specific menopausal symptoms, as well as promote long-term health. Yoga, tai chi, and chi gong are soothing and relaxing and also stimulate the system. Every woman passing through menopause can benefit from these gentle forms of exercise. But vigorous exercise also has its benefits. A good workout that results in shedding a little perspiration energizes the system, speeds the elimination of toxins, dispels angst, and helps keep the heart healthy. Weight-bearing exercise, which includes lifting weights and walking, is perfect for women, as this activity strengthens bones. Add Step 4 to your life, and you'll benefit in many ways. Sports, dance, and physical challenges add richness to life.

Step 5: Stress Management and Menopause

Stress, both physical and emotional, is a well-known trigger of menopausal symptoms. For instance, hot flashes and everyday annoyances often go hand in hand. Step 5 tells you about how the body's reaction to stress can affect crucial aspects of female health, such as hormone production. The adrenal glands, which secrete hormones that govern the stress response, are also involved in producing a significant estrogenic post-menopause. The syntheses of both types of hormones are closely related. When stress places demand on adrenal function, estrogen output declines. This practical step introduces you to the various vitamins and minerals that are depleted by stress. Certain foods replenish these while others consume reserves. Herbs and exercise are valuable tools in managing the stress response. Step 5 explains how to relax by using paced breathing and quiet time to meditate. Experiment with these approaches and find a mix that works for you.

Step 6: Hormone Replacement Therapy

Many problems associated with menopause are due to an imbalance of hormones and reduced production of hormones. The most direct way to address these changes is by supplementing the missing hormones, such as estrogen and progesterone. Of course, you'll need to consult with a physician who can test your current hormone production levels and give you a prescription for the specific hormones and dosages you need. Supplemental hormones are available in many forms, including pills, patches, and creams. The most widely used are synthetic and have a hormone structure different from that which the female body produces. But these days, "natural" hormones are also available, mainly through independent, compounding pharmacies, which customize hormonal therapies based on individual patient's needs. These hormones have the same structure as the body's hormones and often cause fewer side effects. Step 6 helps you sort your way through the products and options to decide if supplemental hormones are for you. Whatever your decision, remember that Step 6 cannot replace Steps 1 through 5.

Check-In with Yourself

The following chapters give you the Six-Step Healthy Menopause Program in depth. You are guaranteed to be exposed to lots of helpful information. Of course, this will do you no good if you don't make use of it. Before you begin reading more, stop a moment and ask yourself how likely you'll be to follow the advice. Your compliance is an essential part of the Healthy Menopause Program! We all have our excuses. Not enough time, not enough money, and so on. A lifetime habit of putting your needs second to others can also keep you from starting this program. Indeed, accomplishing what you say you'd like to do can be difficult, as life is so busy and complex. Circumstances can prevent you from following the Healthy Menopause Program as you might like, but being aware of the usual excuses may help you keep to your plan.

For starters, make a list of your favorite excuses. How can I think about menopause when I am so busy at work? I'm just too tired to start changing what I eat or figuring out new ways to take care of myself. The thought of menopause makes me feel old, and I instead do not think about it. And so on. What reasons do you fall back on, time and again—reasons that seem very real to you? If you hold on to your goal of excellent health passionately enough, you can get past these. You can use menopause to banish your old reliable excuses for the rest of your life as well. Think of how freeing that would be! Most of the recommendations in this program require little additional time or money. Eating nutritious foods doesn't have to cost more. Being better able to manage stress can save you time and energy. If you are worried about feeling overburdened by beginning the program, look for simple ways to start to incorporate the various steps of this program into your life. One change can lead to another. The sooner you start, the sooner you'll benefit.

Chapter 6: Insomnia and Menopause

In case you're in your 40s, and you're similar to a ton of ladies, you've asked yourself, "What on earth is going on with me?" Maybe different circumferences showed up for the time being and will not disappear regardless of the number of crunches you do. Or then again, perhaps you notice yourself sweating. At the same time lying in bed close to your partner, similarly as when you initially got together — except, for now, it occurs in the night when you're not in the sexual act.

Does it appear as though the world has gotten more moronic and that nobody can do things right any longer? Perhaps your touchiness and emotional episodes aren't brought about by the planets being lopsided; possibly it's perimenopause. In this part, we investigate how your hormones work during your reproductive years and how they change as you approach and enter your nonreproductive years.

Vacillations or deviations in your hormone levels generally trigger the physiological, passionate, and mental changes you may see during perimenopause and menopause. Getting good friends with these hormones and finding out about their capacities will not let you control the devastation they appear to unleash. Realizing that your experience is ordinary, however, can alleviate a great deal of stress and vulnerability.

Setting the Stage

Before we begin, we need to set the stage. Menopause isn't a sickness, inadequacy, or disappointment. Nor is it fundamentally going to be tricky for you — each lady's menopause is unique. Menopause is a natural and essential change throughout everyday life. Similarly, as earliest stages, toddlerhood, immaturity, and youthful adulthood, had their difficulties and prizes, so will your menopausal years. Just this time around, you have the maturity, complexity, and assets to find out about and manage what's happening.

You may see and hear clinical terms like estrogen inadequacy, ovarian disappointment, and vaginal decay to portray menopause and its indications. You may even come across them in this book. These terms aren't intended to convey regrettable underlying meanings. They're intended to depict anticipated conditions. You can view menopause as a characteristic change — not an organ disappointment — is a significant initial step to understanding what may be coming up for you and how best to manage any side effect you experience.

Similarly, as ladies aren't put on earth for the sole purpose of bearing kids, your ovaries aren't there to supply eggs. Your ovaries perform two different duties — one as the holder of the seeds of life (oocytes that later form into eggs), and the other as an upkeep specialist. Your ovaries are an essential wellspring of hormones for your entire body. After menopause, your ovaries don't resign; they change professions. At this point, occupied with creating follicles that convey eggs (which deliver loads of estrogen), the ovaries keep producing hormones (however, in a lot more modest sums than previously) to help keep up by and large body capacities. Since the normal future for individuals in the United States is around 80 years, the normal lady spends somewhat more than a large portion of her life discharging and being prolific. And keeping in mind that we live in a culture that puts a great deal of emphasis on these years, the years following menopause can be — and ought to be — similarly as energizing and productive. You can hope to spend a considerable bit of your life simply being a lady. In certain circles, the organization of hormone treatment (HT) has since a long time ago had the standing of being a piece of the fix-a-disappointment way to deal with menopause. Yet, even though we realize that HT can help control indications like hot flushes and vaginal dryness, it's regularly suggested to counter medical problems like coronary illness and breast cancer. The more you think about your own body, about how common hormones (the ones you make yourself) work, and about how substitution hormones (hormone treatment) work, the more ready you'll be to settle on medical care choices customized only for you.

Speedy! What's a hormone, in any case? The majority of us throw this strange word around lovely nonchalantly in our regular daily existences. We indeed use it a ton in this book; however, what does it certainly mean? hormones are intricate synthetic substances that control the delivery or movement of different synthetic substances. The organization in your body that owns and manages these synthetic compounds is known as the endocrine framework.

Connecting your brain and body

Your brain creates the hormones that direct the creation of sex hormones in your ovaries. You may say that the substances delivered by your mind go about as senior administration, coordinating tasks in your ovaries. The hormones in your ovaries are the field supervisors, coordinating functions in the field, which is your whole body. The hormones created by your cerebrum incorporate all activities to the general aim of reproduction.

Follicle-animating hormone (FSH)

At the point when the cerebrum detects that estrogen and progesterone levels have dropped, it shoots out some FSH to the ovaries to advise them to start creating follicles (nutritious sacs that cover the eggs) and begin delivering estrogen.

Luteinizing hormone (LH)

This hormone triggers ovulation. At the point when LH floods, the follicle delivers the egg. The unwanted follicle wrapping, the corpus luteum, secretes progesterone and estrogen.

Understanding estrogen

A woman's body is particularly dynamic. We don't simply create estrogen; we produce three distinct sorts of estrogen:

Estrone (E1): Inactive estrogen transcendent after menopause

Estradiol (E2): Active estrogen

Estriol (E3): Estrogen is created uniquely during pregnancy. Medical people utilize a shorthand framework when alluding to various estrogen levels to avoid disarray (and extensive sentences).

Throughout the book, we utilize the nonexclusive term estrogen to mean every one of the various sorts of estrogen, except if recognizing them is significant for the current conversation.

Estrone (E1)

After menopause, estrone is the transcendent kind of estrogen gushing through your body. Before menopause, your ovaries make estrone. After menopause, your muscle to fat ratio assumes control over the work of making estrone. The more muscle versus fat you have, the more estrone you have. Estrone is principally a saved type of estrogen. Preceding menopause, your ovaries can change estrone over to the dynamic type of estrogen, estradiol. That change just occurs in premenopausal ovaries.

Estradiol (E2)

You may hear specialists or medical caretakers allude to estradiol by its logical name, 17-beta estradiol. However, most people know it as "the great stuff." Before menopause, estradiol is the dominating type of estrogen delivered by your ovaries and utilized all through your body. Estradiol effectively assists with many diverse physical and mental capacities, including keeping up bone thickness and giving your cerebrum information about levels of the sex hormones. After menopause, your ovaries stop the production of estradiol, and that is the point at which you get large numbers of those irritating side effects like hot blazes, palpitations, changes in your skin, bone, hair, and blood vessels, migraines, etc. Your body can change estrone over to estradiol, yet just with completely working ovaries. Your ovaries are easing back down during perimenopause and menopause, and your body doesn't get close to as much estradiol after menopause as it used to during your reproductive years.

Estriol (E3)

The most vulnerable of the three estrogens are estriol, which your placenta delivers just when you're pregnant. The absence of this hormone shows the absence of pregnancy as only the activities in support of a pregnancy can produce this hormone.

Advancing progesterone

Consider progesterone a star moving gestation; it prepares your uterus to house a fertilized egg. A large portion of your progesterone is made after ovulation. If your egg is ready, the placenta assumes control over progesterone creation during the eighth or 10th seven-day stretches of pregnancy. If the egg isn't fertilized, progesterone levels drop. This absence of progesterone triggers your period. Numerous specialists accept that side effects of premenstrual condition (PMS) can be credited to progesterone. When you pine for desserts, you can thank progesterone, feel exhausted, hold water, and get skin break out. Progesterone prepares your body to sustain a pregnancy. How does this work out? At the point when progesterone levels are high, you feel hungry all the more frequently. Progesterone likewise hinders the assimilation interaction so you can retain supplements better; however, that slower absorption cycle can cause you to feel swollen or bloated. Progesterone can cause despair and increase your cholesterol levels. Progesterone likewise has a steadying impact that causes a few ladies to feel quiet and others to feel dormant. It's every one of them a matter of discernment. However, it isn't just in your mind. Progesterone has been discovered to be multiple times more effective than one of the medications utilized in sedation!

Understanding the Stages of Menopause

Menopause, the interminable delay in your periods (menses), is a unique little something that you don't know has occurred until long after it's finished. Like the first occasion when you met your dearest companion: You presumably had no clue that you'd become so close. You possibly acknowledged how unique that event indeed was the point at which you had the option to think back on it. OK, perhaps menopause is anything but a warm-and-fluffy hello card event. However, it is an entry necessary. Is it accurate to say that you are, or would you say you aren't menopausal? You can respond to that question solely after the reality — after you've gone a year without your period. Large numbers of the irritating manifestations allocated to menopause are a lot more terrible preceding menopause in the stage known as perimenopause.

You get both the irritating symptoms (hot flushes, peevishness, mood swings, etc.) and your period. Good for you. In this part, we explain what's happening in your body during the different phases of menopause and disclose how to pin point where you are in the significant change.

Reviewing perimenopause

For some ladies, perimenopause is a notable instance of history repeating itself. Recollect pubescence (ambiguously)? Recollect the crying jags, the emotional episodes, and the "what's up with my skin!" injuries? Indeed, learn to expect the unexpected. They're b-a-a-a-CK. Indeed, your hormones are prepared to unleash havoc on your body, your feelings, and your intellectual capacities. This time around, nonetheless, you're somewhat more astute (you purchased this book, didn't you?), you have experience managing change. You understand that this also will pass. A few specialists prompt ladies who are encountering periods not to stress over "menopausal" manifestations. Yet, you know (since you read it here) that the symptoms people frequently quality to menopause are typically felt as intensely or more in-rigidly during perimenopause. What's more, perimenopause can keep going for a very long time before a lady quits bleeding by and large and turns out to be menopausal. Your situation will be unique! We've seen records that contain many peri-menopausal manifestations. A few ladies breeze through menopause; others make some more complex memories. Try not to expect that because your mom, your sister, your best friend, or the new lady on the Internet menopause message board you've been surfing portrays a severe or strange manifestation that you will encounter same as well.

Encountering intermittent periods

During perimenopause, things change. Suppose you experience your period around the same time as the full moon for a very long time. You could wake up one day and discover that everything has changed and your body has switched on you.

The hormonal shift is because of changes occurring in your ovaries. Your ovaries hold little oocytes (seeds). Every month, a portion of these seeds form into follicles (tiny sacs that contain an egg). A couple of fine strands develop and discharge an egg. That is the point at which you ovulate. The oocytes in your ovaries are held together by a substance called the stroma. The stroma produces testosterone, and the follicles produce estrogen. At the point when you're youthful, you have countless these tiny seeds. As you age, you have fewer roots and more stroma. As the blend of seeds and stroma in your ovary changes, so does hormone creation. Your ovaries decline their production of estrogen; however, keep on delivering testosterone. In some cases, you ovulate during your cycle; here and there, you don't. In some instances, the FSH doesn't get the follicles creating estrogen first thing. Estrogen levels are low toward the start of your cycle when they ought to be high. Your cerebrum reacts to this absence of outfit and passes by sending another flood of FSH (see the "Connecting your mind and body" area prior in this section). At long last, getting the message, your ovaries become somewhat wild and go into two-fold estrogen creation. Directly when you ought to ovulate and delivering

progesterone, your ovaries are simply going to build up a follicle. That implies you will not ovulate when you typically do, and your period will be late. Your Cycle is wrecked. Your estrogen shoots up, and afterward, it drops down. You get hot flushes and perhaps heart palpitations when estrogen plunges. Yet, exactly when you're persuaded that something is genuinely off base and you need to plan a physical check-up, you get your period. Everything gets back to business as usual. You can't help thinking about why you were so stressed and drop the arrangement (if you made one) until the following bizarre thing occurs. This is all fine (perhaps not with you, but rather with Mother Nature) — it's all essential for perimenopause.

Getting enthusiastic

For certain ladies, it's not the rest disturbance, hot flushes, or palpitations that stand out enough to be noticed — it's the emotional episodes. Also, thank heavens for friends and family in that general area to tell us exactly how peevish and undesirable we've been. Welcome to perimenopause.

Overseeing mental miscues

You're as of now acquainted with the jobs hormones play in your psychological deftness and passionate security since you've managed feminine cycles and, at times, pregnancy. At the point when estrogen levels drop, and progesterone levels climbs before your period, you may get those irritating PMS manifestations like fluffy reasoning, mood swings, depression, and fretful rest.

As hormone levels bounce around during perimenopause, these annoying side effects may turn out to be more ordinary. Estrogen assumes a part in dealing with various mental activities. When estrogen levels take a jump during perimenopause, it can be as stressful as managing a boat that occasionally loses its rudder.

Meeting menopause

The beginning of menopause, by definition, happens a year after your last period. Not many ailments utilize a commemoration date as a reason for analysis, yet suitable for us, menopause is one. That is the reason sorting out who's in the club and who's not is so difficult. After menopause, you're postmenopausal (for the remainder of your life). The term postmenopausal hasn't gotten on in like manner utilization (possibly because it's a particularly significant piece). So, we by and large, utilize the term menopause to allude both to menopause and the postmenopausal years.

Taking everything into account, arriving at menopause is just about a non-event. Your ovaries have been easing back down for quite a long while, creating lower and lower estrogen levels and just delivering eggs irregularly. Halting your periods is a consistent result of every one of these changes. A large portion of the indications attributed to menopause, for the most part, starts during perimenopause. Yet, one after the other (to back) long stretches of lower estrogen-creation levels can bring about medical problems that you don't see until menopause Itself has set in. Over the long run, lower estrogen levels (estradiol specifically) add to osteoporosis, cardiovascular issues, and different sicknesses. Because of these conceivable complications sometime down the road, gynaecologists and internists start estimating your tallness, watching out for your cholesterol levels and circulatory strain readings, and checking your way of life propensities (like exercise and diet) as you approach midlife.

Menopause is an ideal opportunity to survey your eating regimen, practice schedule, and undesirable propensities (smoking or extreme liquor utilization, for instance). In your previous life, your body was excessively lenient. During menopause, your will not make allowance for your dietary excesses. You need to sit up in the knowledge that you will pay (maybe heavily) for every unhealthy bite. During menopause, putting on weight is more straightforward, and losing it is more difficult. What's more, getting a decent night's rest and awakening feeling revived and prepared to face the day isn't just about as simple as it used to be. Make some solid goals and stick with them so you don't end up saying, similar to writer Eubie Blake said when he turned 100, "if I'd realized I was going to live this long, I'd have cared more for myself."

Chapter 7: Sex and Menopause

Bravo for life's little paradoxes. You may find that at about a similar time your children are proceeding onward (and out), you at long last have the time (and the money) for those heartfelt ends of the week; your primary care physician gives you the green light to throw your contraception; your body is prepared to make whoopie, yet your sex organs are planning for retirement. Or then again, you may find that your organs are as yet willing, yet your hormones are most certainly not. Then again, you may expect interest in and limit concerning extraordinary sex to decline, to find that menopause is the best thing that consistently happened to your sexual relationship. Simply don't accept that the desperate forecasts about the loss of drive and dewy newness offering an approach to lack of engagement and dryness are the standard for everybody. Loads of ladies discover sex after menopause to be better than anyone might have expected.

Doubtlessly however, that sex changes after menopause — your hormonal movements have repercussions for your genitals just as your moving parts. There's additionally a lot of annoying social unreasonableness to manage — a dreadful parcel of people holds to the possibility that ladies of a particular age should not be attractive or sexual. In this section, we'll discuss why you shouldn't say farewell to your sexual coexistence presently, why you actually should be cautious about conception prevention (and why it may not be past the point of no return for a child if that is the place where your heart lies), and propose a few different ways to keep the home flames copying as you approach and enter menopause.

Taking a look at Menopause and its effects on your libido

Menopause opens another section in your life, so it's nothing unexpected that the sexual you change. Much of the time, the improvements are. Even though there will never have been a clinical justification for you to go without sex during your period, most ladies and their Partners shun sex for those days. Since those feminine periods have taken off (or are at any rate pressing for the excursion), you have more freedom for sex. Also, recall how you generally appeared to get your period when you were on holiday, regardless of how well you arranged? Presently you can mess about to your heart's content without checking and twofold checking for those red circles on your schedule. The cantankerousness, issues, and headache that portrayed quite a bit of your period presently level out into a kinder and gentler articulation of you. Sex drive frequently reduces with age. Most research examinations have tracked down that little change in sexual action happens between 45 and 55. In any case, somewhere in the range of 55 and 65, sexual act eases back. Also, however, ladies in their 60s may not participate in sex as frequently as they did in their more youthful years; no change happens in the recurrence of climax or the degree of sexual happiness. Thus, you may not do it as regularly. However, sex is similarly fulfilling. (A fascinating note: Research shows that movement with sexual accomplices regularly endures well before ladies stop stroking off.)

Quality doesn't need to decrease with quantity!

The fluctuating hormones that portray menopause and perimenopause unquestionably affect your sex drive. Be ready for a steady increment — or a progressive reduction — in your sex drive. You may not know about any change whatsoever. Yet, most menopausal ladies experience at any rate brief times of a higher-or lower-than-regular sex drive.

Leaving your sentiments alone, talk about sex.

Nobody knows your body better than you, so focus on it. Since each lady encounters menopause somewhat differently, your clinical consultant may not be conversant with what's typical for you — and what appears to be changed to you. Figure out how to confide in yourself and discuss transparently with your PCP.

This guidance goes twofold for changes in your sex drive (want to engage in sexual relations). Numerous doctors and GYN disregard sexual issues while treating perimenopausal and menopausal ladies. So, it's significant that you raise the case if your PCP doesn't. Here are some valuable clues for conversing with your PCP:

Specialists have heard everything; don't feel humiliated about your questions or concerns. If you don't feel great talking about sex and sexuality with your primary care physician, fine one with whom you are comfortable.

Bring up your issues from the get-go in the arrangement. Pause for a minute just after the "Howdy, how are you getting along today" part to raise the issue by saying something, for example, " . . . furthermore, there's another issue that we need to settle before I leave today." Waiting until you're going the way to raise a delicate issue occurs so regularly that specialists have a name for the marvel: "the door handle second."

Keep a journal of any agony, inconvenience, or release you experience identified with sex. Track things, for example, how long it keeps going, what movement may have caused the issue, and the level and nature of torment you felt.

Sexual responsiveness is a characteristic cycle, not a privilege saved for extraordinary individuals. If you're encountering problematic changes in your sexual drive after menopause, be immediate with your primary care physician. The issue might be hormonal (low testosterone levels) or other clinical explanations behind the change.

If your primary care physician can preclude clinical issues that may be meddling with your sexual fulfilment yet doesn't appear to be open to assist you with pursuing an answer, request a reference to a subject matter expert — for this situation, an accredited sex specialist.

Turning up the heat

The more significant part of all menopausal ladies keeps up a similar degree of sexual interest after menopause as in the past. Indeed, you may feel less hindered when the chance of pregnancy no longer lingers in your mind. After you have gone an entire year without a period, you can be more liberated to have unprotected Sex at any time you want.

The renowned sex research group of Masters and Johnson demonstrated to the world that sexual hunger isn't attached to estrogen levels (even though you may require a little grease to make sex agreeable after estrogen decreases). It's the androgens (male sex hormones like testosterone) delivered by your ovaries for the duration of your life that keep your sex drive running. Even after menopause (when your ovaries have escaped the estradiol and progesterone-favorable to duction game), your ovaries continue creating androgens.

Suppose you have intercourse with more than one accomplice during or after menopause. In that case, you need to rehearse safe sex to avoid getting an explicitly sent infection or AIDS. Even though men don't go through menopause, their testosterone levels steadily decay after 40. The physiological changes don't occur incidentally. Over the long haul, men will see that it takes more time for them to get an erection. They aren't stimulated as effectively, which might be uplifting news for a lady who appreciates foreplay. Ladies whose accomplices endure untimely discharge can cheer. That issue may disappear, and men acquire enduring force as they age. Regardless of whether you're having fewer periods (or maybe you haven't had one in months), don't surrender your anti-conception medication until you've been without periods for an entire year. During perimenopause, your hormone levels and the possibility of ovulation are wildly unusual. It's improbable. However, you could have a hormonally hot month and end up pregnant.

Managing a reduced sex drive

An excellent mental self-view and grown-up way of life, for the most part, incorporate fulfilling and safe sexual movement. However, many (yet not all) ladies are disappointed by a declining want for sex during and after menopause. Understanding the science behind a declining drive can help achieve an answer. Your sex drive can decrease sooner than you'd like for a few reasons. Some are mental or enthusiastic — if your confidence falls in light of changes in your day-to-day existence or body, you may need to address that issue before you can track down your old drive. A portion of the reasons are physical — complicated sex isn't anything to search forward to.

Furthermore, some are hormonal — your hormones are changing. If you'd prefer to keep up your sex drive, your hormones should be adjusted. Speaking with your PCP is considerably more important if you've encountered early menopause. If your primary care physician trifles with your interests in sex, track down another specialist. You will not have the option to get pregnant after menopause. However, you can, in any case, have a hot and solid sexual life.

Changing your demeanor

It's challenging to feel affectionate when you're depressed. Menopause, in itself, doesn't make you depressed, yet consider the sorts of things occurring during these years:

Children venturing out from home

Parents maturing and requiring nearer consideration

You or your life partner retiring

Add to these difficulties the common issues of keeping a positive relationship and simply adapting to a speedy world. Presently, the one thing that used to be dependable, your body, is likewise changing at a quicker speed than it has in a long while. Is anyone surprised that sex is the last thing at the forefront of your thoughts?

Yet, suppose the absence of actual flash disturbs you. In that case, you need to dispose of the enthusiastic stressors before you can anticipate that your libido should kick in. It might simply require some investment in yourself. Set aside some effort to get an activity program going. Strolling consistently without help from anyone else or with a companion can do a lot to lessen pressure. Talk with companions, a specialist, your beautician, or a pastor about your difficulties. Likewise, make sure to raise your uneasiness or depression when you converse with your internist or gynaecologist.

Ensuring that menopausal sex isn't a painful experience

Hormonal changes can make the vaginal covering more slender, more delicate, and more defenseless from tearing and create less grease. Vaginal connective tissue likewise turns out to be less malleable, and sensitive spots become less reactive. The result of this organic mix is that intercourse may get painful and stressful.

Sexual action that used to cause incredible delight would now cause torment. The possibility of the distress may make you need to get a migraine or wipe out your sock cabinet when your partner makes loving advances. However, everything isn't lost. You can mitigate difficult intercourse in an assortment of ways:

Maintain an active and functioning sexual life.

Ordinary sexual action keeps blood circling in your vulva and eases back the drying cycle. So maintaining a functioning sexual life may help you stay away from the torment related to dry vaginal tissues. This is undoubtedly one of those "use it or You lose it" circumstances.

Converse with your accomplice about the touchier you. Most men don't know that hormonal changes trigger changes in your vulva and vagina. Disclose to your accomplice that you two need to sort out new room methodologies that can be commonly fulfilling.

Take an uncompromising stance

This is an incredible opportunity to try different things with new situations for sex. We're not going to disclose to you which pages in the Kama Sutra to consult; however, lady on-top positions may give you more power over your solace.

Utilize an ointment during intercourse to help keep things moving

Lubrication can bear the cost of long stretches of relational joy. A few ladies and their partners make ointment application a piece of foreplay. Water-based lubricants, like Astroglide, are better for vaginal linings. Stay away from petrol-based items. Now and then, ladies experience everyday inconvenience because of vaginal dryness — not simply during sex. If you're one of them, you can consistently utilize different ointments to mitigate this aggravation.

Try not to utilize estrogen cream as a sexual ointment. The estrogen cream can be consumed by your accomplice and cause issues. At any rate, one instance of Breast cancer has been recorded in a man since his better half utilized vaginal estrogen cream as an ointment. It's critical to peruse the guidelines!

It's not the estrogen!

Numerous reports and books make a tremendous arrangement about how no logical proof connections relating estrogen levels to a declining sex drive. These publications, at that point, take the jump toward wrongly presuming that hormones have nothing to do with grit. Although the estrogen may not assume the choosing part in the drive guideline, the harmony between estrogen and testosterone likely affects it. This subject is somewhat dubious, so we need to give you the two sides of the contention. On one side are researchers who infer that enhancing your testosterone during menopause expands your moxie. On the opposite side are the ones who accept that the science doesn't exist to show that testosterone is either protected or compelling for ladies who complain of low sex drive. Testosterone is delivered typically by ladies' ovaries and affects your drive, state of mind, imperativeness, feeling of prosperity, bone, and muscle. Yet, even before menopause, your body hinders its creation of testosterone. After menopause, you produce about half as much testosterone as you created during your reproductive years. So, it's not uncommon for your moxie to decrease if your testosterone levels are deficient. You would prefer not to have an excessive amount of testosterone either — it can cause breast and liver cancer. In addition, an excessive amount of testosterone compared with estrogen can release the impacts of testosterone that estrogen had been monitoring, like beard growth, expanded moxie, reallocation of muscle to fat ratio (it moves to the center of your body), and skin breaks out. A few specialists avoid recommending testosterone as a feature of hormone treatment (HT) because they're apprehensive about disturbing the estrogen/testosterone equilibrium and causing upsetting results. The stunt, if you're taking HT with testosterone, is to keep testosterone levels sufficiently high to stay away from one bunch of products (counting low charisma) and then offset with different hormones to stay away from another arrangement of products (beard growth or skin break out, for instance). Those people in the logical and clinical networks who see testosterone as a commendable treatment for moxie issues accept that exorbitantly high doses of testosterone bring about the awful results felt by certain ladies. Defenders of testosterone use recommend utilizing low measurements and keeping balance between the degrees of testosterone and estrogen.

Chatting straightforwardly about Testosterone

Remember that men, just as ladies, experience declining drive as they age! In case you're seeing changes in your sexual relationship, take solace in the fact that your accomplice's hormones are evolving as well. Men produce significantly more testosterone than ladies, and however, when they arrive at 40, their testosterone levels start declining. In any case, most men don't see a noticeable change in their charisma for about an additional ten years. Around 50 or thereabouts, the drop in testosterone makes men quit having psychogenic (erections from simply contemplating sex). Men who could have an erection immediately find that it's somewhat more complicated (no play on words intended) to get things going. Along these lines, in case you're concerned because your accomplice isn't seeking after you like he used to, your menopause may not be at the core of the matter. Your accomplice might be going through hormonal changes of his own, even though his transformation isn't just about as sensational as yours. You may even find that his progressions are viable with yours. It might take him longer to arrive at climax than it used to, giving both of you more opportunity for long, moderate, open to lovemaking.

Chapter 8: The ideal dietary plan for a woman during the perimenopausal transition

Because nutrient-rich foods provide a foundation for good health, eating nourishing foods makes up the second step of the Healthy Menopause Program. As fundamental as eating well is too good health, diet is not usually emphasized in medical protocols. Suppose you consult a conventional physician about lessening symptoms of menopause. In that case, you are most likely to be offered hormone replacement therapy (HRT) as the first line of defense. One significant advantage of using food to prevent menopause symptoms is that food is not likely to cause side effects. The same cannot be said of hormone replacement therapy. And even if you take supplemental hormones, you still have to eat. Find out all you can learn about foods for menopause and those that should be avoided, starting with the following information.

The Standard Diet and Menopause

Many of the most commonly eaten foods can undermine your health and make your passage through menopause more difficult. The great majority of meals contain some form of refined wheat and refined white sugar. The average American consumes approximately 155 pounds of sugar each year. Vegetables are scarce, and meats and fried foods are ample. To make matters worse, the meal is often washed down with cola and topped off with caffeinated coffee to rev up the system after this energy-depleting repast. Nutritionist Vesanto Melina, R.D., sees the effects of such a diet in her practice. As she reports: The women I consult with who have been eating an average American diet have a fair amount of trouble with menopause. But it's another story with women who are more of the healthy food types. They've been exercising, and they aren't overly fast, and because of what they have been eating, their bodies are prepared and are not toxic. When it comes to menopause, these women are just cruising through.

Sugar

When you eat sugars, including refined white sugar, maple syrup, and honey, your body metabolizes these to glucose. This simple sugar circulates in the blood. Glucose is a source of energy and the only fuel that the brain can use. For normal functioning, you need a relatively steady level of blood glucose. In susceptible individuals, the ability to manage glucose levels can diminish with age. It may be that problems attributed to menopause at midlife also involve glucose metabolism. Low blood sugar stresses the system and can trigger various symptoms, including anxiety, fatigue, poor memory, and even hot flashes. As an average blood glucose level is restored, the effects are just as dramatic, with evidence of increased energy and mental clarity.

Steadying Blood Glucose

You can do much to steady your blood sugar levels by following these simple guidelines:

•Be sure to eat three meals a day at regular intervals, beginning with breakfast.

•Have a snack between meals if you feel your blood sugar dropping.

•Be sure to include carbohydrates, proteins, and fats in your diet. Each of these food groups provide energy at a different rate. By eating all three simultaneously, you help ensure that you will have an even supply of blood sugar over about 3 hours. Carbohydrates

break down in about 1½ hours, protein after 2 to 2½ hours, and fats
after 3 hours.

Fibre

Estrogens produced by the body eventually leave the body via the
intestinal tract. As they pass through the large intestine, some may
combine with other compounds and, in this form, eventually be
reabsorbed back into the system. However, fibre intake appears to
help control the level of estrogens in the blood by pro- moving its
excretion. A diet high in fibre may help reduce symptoms of
menopause associated with high levels of estrogen, such as anxiety
and the risk of breast cancer, which is also related to this type of
hormone imbalance. Colas contain sugar, caffeine, and phosphoric
acid, a cocktail of substances that can undermine female health.
Besides the effects of sugar already described, the caffeine in cola
stresses the adrenal glands, an essential source of sex hormones
after menopause. Overworked adrenal glands appear to be
involved in hormonal imbalances that can bring on menopausal
symptoms. (Caffeinated coffee and teas have the same effect.) And
phosphoric acid can increase phosphorus levels in the bloodstream,
causing calcium to be pulled from the skeletal system, thereby
setting the stage for osteoporosis to develop.

Improving Your Diet

If you've been skipping breakfast and having fast-food lunches,
with a sudden improvement in the diet, you may feel better in just
days. Hot flashes brought on by having a Danish pastry and a
strong cup of caffeinated coffee abate as soon as the offending
foods are cut from the diet. However, fully restoring your
hormonal health and vitality, and general well-being may take 2 to
3 months or even longer. You need to increase your body's stores
of vitamins, minerals, and other nutrients. Once you build up your
nutrient reserves and begin to feel better, you may be tempted to

return to your old ways. You may have a grace period during which it's easy to think that it doesn't matter what you eat and that you are through the worst of menopause anyway. But continue your previous habits for a week or two, and menopausal symptoms are likely to recur—it's an excellent way to test how bad some foods can make you feel!

Whole Foods

Eating for menopause can be a pleasure. The freshest, most natural, and beautifully colored ingredients are just what you need. Golden squash, ruby-red berries, the season's best peaches, and figs, glistening fresh fish, raw nuts and seeds, and frilly herbs are on the menu! These foods and others like them are rich sources of the many nutrients essential for menopause presented in Chapter 4. These ingredients all have something in common. They are whole foods—foods with all their parts, such as beets plus their tops, potatoes with their skins. These foods are also unrefined, unprocessed, and free of added hormones, artificial flavors, and coloring agents. You can find whole foods at your regular supermarket, in natural food stores, and at farmers' markets. The price of fresh food can sometimes seem expensive, especially if it is organic. Still, such foods cost less, pound for pound, than foods that have been refined, altered, and elaborately packaged and advertised. For some food products, nearly 75% of each dollar you spend may go to the manufacturer's costs, not the food itself.

Traditional Foods versus the Modern Diet

From the Mediterranean coast and Africa, women in many parts of the world These various populations fare better because traditional and whole foods still make up a significant part of their diet. Meals are made from staples such as lentils, whole grains, fresh nuts and seeds, and seasonal fruits and vegetables. Fish is eaten far more frequently than in North America, and red meat and poultry are consumed in smaller portions. Particularly in less developed countries and in more rural areas, meals are likely to be made up of simple fare. People cook with ingredients that are grown locally and are often less processed. Consequently, such foods are likely to contain higher levels of nutrients and fewer harmful hormones.

Plant Foods to the Rescue

Eating a vegetarian or mostly vegetarian diet is associated with fewer menopausal symptoms. As women's health specialist Susan M. Lark, M.D., recommends, "For optimal health, women need to eat a plant foods-based diet, emphasizing whole grains, legumes including beans and peas, raw seeds and nuts, and lots of fruits and vegetables. And if a woman wants to eat meat, fish is a better choice than red meat or poultry." Dr. Lark continues, "There is evidence that women who follow this type of program can reduce and prevent menopause symptoms. These foods are great sources of phytoestrogens, minerals such as calcium and magnesium, and essential fatty acids, all-important for a woman's health." A survey conducted for *Prevention* magazine in 1993 supp orts these recommendations. The research, headed by Fredi Kronenberg, PhD, director of menopause research at the Center for Women's Health at Columbia-Presbyterian Medical Centre, New York City, assessed the relationship of menopausal symptoms to diet and found that women who were vegetarians or who ate mostly vegetarian foods re- ported significantly fewer symptoms than women who only occasionally if ever had vegetarian meals. In addition, soy foods were associated with fewer symptoms. One explanation for these apparent benefits may be that vegetarian and eat soy live a healthier lifestyle in general. Another answer is that such a diet supplies many phytoestrogens, which help even out hormones that can bring on symptoms when out of balance. (See Chapter 4 for more on phytoestrogens.) According to a study published in the *British Med*

ical Journal in 1990, researchers in Melbourne, Australia, found
that supplementing women's diets with estrogenic foods resulted in
signs of an estrogen response. (For experimental purposes, this is
measured by microscopic examination of vaginal cells. The
vaginal wall thickens as the amount of estrogen in the system
increases.) In the study, estrogenic foods made up about 10% of
the women's diet. However, as the study points out, estrogenic
plants provide 50% of the calorie's women consume each day in
some parts of the world. A diet so abundant in phytoestrogens may
play a significant role in diminishing menopausal symptoms.

Organic Foods

Organic food is grown without pesticides, herbicides, or hormone
fertilizers on land that has been free of hormones for at least three
preceding years. Fertilizers and mulches must consist only of
animal and vegetable matter. "Certified" organic is a guarantee that
an independent organization has inspected some combination
of the produce, the soil, and the grower's methods and has made
sure that they meet the established standard. Although plant food
can be only as nutrient-rich as the soil in which it was grown, there
is some evidence that organic foods may contain higher levels of
vitamins and minerals. An often-cited study is "Organic Foods vs
Supermarket Foods: Element Levels," published in 1993 in
Applied *Nutrition*. Organic pears, apples, potatoes, and wheat
sampled over two years contained an average of 90% more
nutrients than similar commercial nonorganic foods. This nutrient
bonus, often available in organic foods, is just what women need
as they approach menopause. Insecticides such as endosulfan and
methoxychlor that are widely used on crops are classed as
estrogen-like compounds. Whereas the body quickly breaks
down phytoestrogens naturally present in plant foods, synthetic
estrogens tend to build up in the blood and fatty tissue over time.
The effect of these hormones may be sufficient to upset a woman's

hormone balance and help trigger menopausal symptoms. There may also be a link between synthetic estrogens and breast cancer, a further reason to shop for organic foods. Although some dangerous pesticides have been banned in North America, these same pesticides continue to be sold to farmers in other countries, especially Central and South America.

Crops treated with this return to North America and are sold in grocery stores. Such produce makes up about 10% of the total intake of fruits and vegetables. This figure may be even higher in northern regions during the winter months when local crops are not available. Some toxins in the environment, although not estrogenic, are capable of interfering with the reproductive system. Dioxin, an unintentional by-product of many industrial processes involving chlorine, is a known human carcinogen and can cause severe reproductive problems. Dioxin is in commonly eaten foods such as beef, milk and other dairy products, chicken, and pork, and to a lesser extent, fish and eggs. It is fat-soluble and moves up the food chain. Fortunately, more stores are making organic foods available. If the produce buyer or butcher in your neighborhood market has not yet begun offering this choice, take the initiative and explain that you want more female-friendly foods!

The Best Foods for Menopause

Within every food category, from grains to beverages, certain foods are especially abundant in nutrients for menopause. Take a look at the following items and begin to include the recommended foods in your shopping list.

Whole Grains

Whole grains are a source of vitamin E, one of the essential nutrients for discouraging hot flashes. They supply B vitamins that nourish the nervous system and help steady emotions. In addition, because whole grains are digested more slowly than refined grains, these foods are less likely to trigger abrupt changes in blood sugar and trigger symptoms. When grain is refined, the wheat germ is removed along with the healthy oils, B vitamins, and vitamin E. When this refined grain is used to make bread, manufacturers enrich the grain. Still, only some of the original nutrients are returned. Refined wheat, compared with whole wheat, contains less vitamin E, magnesium, calcium, copper, iron, phosphorus, potassium, selenium, zinc, and even lower amounts of some of the B vitamins enriched. Refining also re- moves fibre, which helps balance hormones.

GRAIN PRESCRIPTION

Be sure to eat various grains such as oats and millet and grains such as quinoa, a staple of early civilizations in South America. And enjoy buckwheat, which is not a grain but the seed of an herb. Buckwheat supplies estrogenic bioflavonoids. In eastern European countries and Russia, buckwheat is eaten as kasha, and Japanese cook with soba noodles made of buckwheat. Choose from among the following: oats, barley, rye, brown rice, whole-wheat couscous, bulgur wheat, millet, cornmeal, quinoa, Amaranthe, Kamut.

SHOPPING FOR WHOLE GRAINS

Look for labels that specifically state "whole grain," which means that the flour was not refined. Whole wheat is not whole grain. Whole-wheat bread usually has as its first ingredient some form of refined wheat flour. These days, you can find whole-grain bagels, English muffins, and croissants. You can also find whole-grain hot breakfast cereal in natural food stores, such as cream of whole wheat, cream of brown rice, and cream of buckwheat. Some raw food stores even carry whole-grain croutons and ready-made bread crumbs.

Legumes

Legumes, that is, beans, lentils, and peas, are a mineral-rich, low-fat source of protein, which is just what you want in your diet as you approach midlife. Your body needs the minerals to help maintain strong bones and manage stress. Reducing your fat intake can help you curb the weight gain that your sex hormone production changes. Beans are also high in water-soluble fiber, which can help lower cholesterol.

LEGUME PRESCRIPTION

Beans are eaten less frequently than years ago. To increase your intake, include them in soups and salads. Soybeans are exceptionally high in phytoestrogens. Choose from among the following: navy beans, pinto beans, black beans, lima beans, lentils, black-eyed peas, chickpeas, soybeans.

Vegetables and Fruit

One of the Dietary Guidelines for Americans is to eat at least five servings a day of fruits and vegetables. As Hugh Riordan, M.D., says, "It's generally thought that if you were to eat the recommended minimum of five servings a day, you might indeed have good levels of vitamins and minerals in your body. But the current estimate is that less than 9% of the population eats this much. This means that probably a lot of women begin menopause missing important nutrients that they need." To increase your intake, snack on fruit at work. In restaurants, order a salad that includes a variety of vegetables. At home, cook vegetable soups. When you shop for produce, invest in the best quality you can find. Whenever possible, buy fresh local fruits and vegetables. Local produce can be more nutritious and is less likely to be treated with preservatives used to keep produce new while being transported long distances to market. It's also expected to be higher in nutrients, which the rigors of shipping can destroy. And suppose you buy local produce at a farmers' market. In that case, you have the opportunity to talk directly to the grower and check whether the crop was sprayed with pesticides.

VEGETABLE PRESCRIPTION

Some vegetables are exceptionally high in nutrients that support health during and post-menopause. However, the best advice is to eat various vegetables, which can supply you with a range of nutrients. Choose from among the following: red onions, asparagus, artichokes, winter squash, broccoli, green beans, celery, sweet red peppers, garlic, parsley, tomatoes, kale.

THE DIRTY DOZEN

The Environmental Working Group (EWG), a non-profit environmental research organization, assembled a list of 12 fruits and vegetables that have been found to contain the highest levels of pesticides. The EWG estimates that you can cut your health risk from pesticides by about 50% by avoiding these foods or choosing organically grown varieties. Take a look at the following list, which also gives you alternatives that supply some of the same nutrients.

1.Strawberries. *Alternatives:* blackberries, raspberries, blueberries, citrus fruit such as oranges and grapefruit, watermelon, U.S.-grown cantaloupe, and kiwi

2.Bell peppers. *Alternatives:* romaine lettuce, broccoli, peas, tomat oes, carrots, broccoli, asparagus, brussels sprouts

3.Spinach. *Alternatives:* asparagus, brussels sprouts, romaine lettuc e, broccoli

4.U.S.-
grown cherries. *Alternatives:* blueberries, blackberries, oranges, gr apefruit, kiwi, U.S.-grown cantaloupe

5.Peaches. *Alternatives:* nectarines, red or pink grapefruit, oranges, tangerines, watermelon, U.S.–grown cantaloupe

6.Mexican-grown cantaloupe. *Alternatives:* U.S.-grown cantaloupe, watermelon

7.Celery. *Alternatives:* radishes, carrots, broccoli, romaine lettuce

8.Apples. *Alternatives:* citrus including oranges, grapefruit, and tangerines, nectarines, bananas, pears, kiwi, watermelon, U.S.-grown cantaloupe

9.Apricots. *Alternatives:* red or pink grapefruit, oranges, tangerines, nectarines, U.S.-grown cantaloupe, watermelon

10.Green beans. *Alternatives:* broccoli, peas, cauliflower, potatoes, asparagus, brussels sprouts

11.Grapes from Chile. *Alternatives:* U.S.-grown grapes available in season from May to December

12.Cucumbers. *Alternatives:* carrots, broccoli, radishes, romaine lettuce

Meat and Poultry

Although many women in menopause feel best eating a vegetarian or mostly vegetarian diet, animal protein, including meat and poultry, can have a place in a menopause diet. These foods supply protein, which your body requires daily since protein is not stored. According to the U.S. Department of Agriculture's Food Guide Pyramid, you need two to three servings a day of protein food from various sources: meat, poultry, fish, dry beans, eggs, and nuts. (Not included in the protein section of the pyramid are vegetables and grains, which are also good sources of protein.) Recommended portion sizes for meat are smaller than you might think: only

4 ounces. Four ounces of hamburger is the size of a pack of cards—hardly the Amer- can standard for a serving of steak! However, such modest portions are just what is needed if you top a salad with strips of grilled chicken breast or add chunks of beef to a bean and vegetable soup—both excellent menu choices for menopause. Choosing lean cuts of meat is also essential to help manage weight and limit the intake of saturated fats. Thin and round cuts of meat, such as pork loin and white-meat chicken rather than dark meat, have less fat. Visible fat should be trimmed from meat and poultry. Meat and poultry are good sources of B vitamins and many minerals needed for good health.

In particular, meat is an excellent source of vitamin B12 and energ y nutrient essential for normal functioning of the nervous system, and iron, an oxygen-carrying component of blood. Heavy menstrual flow can cause iron to be- to come depleted, causing fatigue.

You may also want to schedule *when* you eat meat according to yo ur menstrual cycle. Red meat, and to a lesser degree, pork and poultry contain arachidonic acid. This substance can lead to menstrual cramps, which occur in some women as they develop irregular periods during perimenopause. If you suffer from menstrual cramps, stay away from meat and dairy foods for at least a few days pre- ceding and during your menstrual cycle.

CHOOSE "CLEAN" MEATS

Go out of your way to buy meat raised without added hormones. These hormones can alter the balance of your hormones and may contribute to menopausal symptoms. Look for meats that are labeled "residue-free."

Fish and Shellfish

Seafood, including fish and shellfish, is an excellent source of minerals. Seafood supplies iodine, magnesium, manganese, copper, phosphorus, and notably selenium. A trace mineral is lacking in the standard North American diet. Selenium boosts the benefits of vitamin E, a nutrient vital for menopausal health. Seafood is also a source of fat-soluble vitamins A, D, and E. In addition, seafood is an excellent source of omega-3 fatty acids— quality fats that play a vital role in female health post-menopause. Omega-3 helps maintain vaginal health, skin quality, and good memory. Richer-tasting, oilier fish contain

the highest amounts, for example, salmon, tuna, mackerel, herring, and anchovies. Caviar is also a superb source! Make an effort to eat fish two or three times a week to benefit from this exceptionally healthy source of nutrients. However, eating seafood more frequently than this can have its drawbacks. Because of polluted waters, seafood can contain heavy metals and other toxins. Limit your exposure by eating a variety of seafood, and eat smaller fish lower on the food chain and are less likely to concentrate toxins, and eat offshore fish such as sole, cod, and tuna.

Fats and Oils

Fat is feared because overeating can put on pounds, especially post-menopause when most women gain weight. Indeed, the average North American consumes too many calories from fat, about 40% of calories rather than the 30% recommended by the American Heart Association. However, quality fats are an essential part of a healthy diet. Fat helps the body stay warm. Fat insulates the nerves and provides cushioning to protect organs. And fat is the raw material from which hormones are made. Health does not depend on the quantity of fat consumed but on the quality. The healthiest fats and oils on the market are:

Extra-virgin olive oil

Unrefined safflower oil

Unrefined sesame oil

Flaxseed oil

Organic, unsalted butter

Monounsaturated fats, such as olive oil, are associated with lower rates of heart disease. In contrast, saturated fats, found in butter and coconut oil, can clog arteries. When eaten in excess, polyunsaturated fats, such as canola, safflower, and grape- seed oil fall somewhere in between, lowering low-density lipoprotein (LDL), the bad cholesterol, but also high-density lipoprotein (HDL), the good cholesterol. Some of these kinds of fat have a place in a healthy diet, emphasizing monounsaturated and polyunsaturated.

Reach for unrefined oils

Select oils that include the word *unrefined* on the label. They still c ontain their original vitamins and minerals, chlorophyll, and such compounds as phytoestrogens, destroying or removing the refining process. The only widely sold unrefined oil is extra-virgin olive oil; however, you can also find unrefined safflower oil, a polyunsaturated oil, in natural food stores. Another unrefined oil that deserves to be a staple in your kitchen is flaxseed oil. It is a rich source of omega-3 fatty acids. Flaxseed oil is very fragile and will become rancid when exposed to heat, light, or air.

For this reason, it is sold
in opaque plastic bottles and kept in the refrigerator section in store s. *Never heat flaxseed oil.* Add it to food after the food has been co oked and placed on a serving plate. Or use it in salad dressing,

mixed with extra-virgin olive oil. Be sure to make the dressing fresh each time you have some.

Butter is better

While butter is saturated fat, it is stable and not readily broken down by light, oxygen, or heat. Butter is minimally processed and still contains the natural antioxidants vitamin E and selenium. The most refined quality butter is unsalted and organic. In contrast, margarine is made from highly refined oil heated to high temperatures, generating trans-fatty acids. A trans-fatty acid has a strange twist in its structure. In your body, trans-fatty acids can increase blood cholesterol levels and blood fat levels, both risk factors for heart disease. They can also interfere with sugar metabolism, the immune response, and pregnancy and may even be a factor in cancer.

When to Begin—the Sooner the Better

If you are not yet in menopause or have just begun to notice changes in your body, you can do yourself a big favor by starting to eat well. The number of symptoms you may experience at menopause depends on your state of health when menopause begins. As Russell Jaffee, M.D., points out, "The difficulties women experience at menopause are linked to their nutritional deficiencies, not their chronology." Closely allied with nutrition is the use of herbs to create health during menopause. Step 3 of the Healthy Menopause Program shows you how to make use of herbs to ease symptoms.

Herbs and Menopause

The Healthy Menopause Program relies for the most part on natural means of healing and achieving well-being. One of the most critical aspects of this program is the use of herbs. Many herbs have medicinal effects, just like pharmaceutical drugs, but fundamentally they too are food. Think of them as a source of nourishment, just like bananas and pumpkin seeds! Producers of herbal remedies use raw materials derived from cultivated plants or those collected in the wild. Herbs are not necessarily derived from natural herbs. Herbal medicine also uses roots, leaves, seeds, and the bark of shrubs, vines, and trees. Some are taken in capsule form like any prescription. Some can be added to everyday meals or enjoyed brewed as teas. Drugs consist of isolated ingredients. In contrast, medicinal plants contain a variety of healing substances.

For this reason, herbalists will often use the whole plant in treating a patient. The seemingly fewer valuable components work synergistically with the active ingredients to deliver a far gentler form of healing than pharmaceuticals offer. Plants contain two fundamental types of compounds: active ingredients, Chemists' study and drug manufacturers' research to develop new products, and all the other substances and mixtures primarily ignored by modern medicine. It is the totality of these that herbalists rely on to promote healing and health. The supporting compounds may help the body more easily benefit from an herb or temper the action of a very potent plant hormone, helping to prevent side effects. Some substances may even prevent overdosing by triggering nausea when an individual has taken more of a plant than the system can tolerate. Herbs can be effective treatments and tonics, thanks to their primary active ingredients and these secondary compounds.

Special Compounds

Healing plants and herbs contain a range of health-supportive substances.   One category is *volatile oils*, including alkaloids, bitters, flavonoids, glycosides, an d tannins. Another group is the *steroidal saponins*. These compoun ds affect the production and balance of hormones that are also steroids. Saponins are present in various herbs used traditionally for female health, such as black cohosh, blue cohosh, ginseng, false unicorn root, squaw vine, fenugreek, wild yam, and liquorice. Drugs have a single effect, whereas herbs have a complexity of actions, which explains why they can treat only opposite conditions. Herbs that contain phytohormones can be used as a remedy for low estrogen as well as low progesterone. If using herbal medicine seems to you a bit too folksy, even risky, consider this: At least 25% of all modern pharmaceutical drugs are derived from herbs. In addition, the classic herbs used to treat such problems as hot flashes and mood swings have a legacy of success that spans centuries. Native American women relied on black cohosh to balance sex hormones and reduce menopausal symptoms. This herb is still prescribed for menopause today.

Herbal Remedies Can Be Taken in Many Forms

One option is to buy dried plants and make up your preparations to save money. You can even purchase empty gelatin capsules and fill these yourself with the herbs you plan to take. However, such a hands-on approach takes time and effort and is not recommended for newcomers to herbal medicine. Start with readymade, high-quality herbal products such as whole herbs, herbal extracts and tinctures, and herbs in capsules.

•You can prepare a cup of healing herbal tea right in your kitchen by brewing the dried leaves, stems, or flowers of a plant such as mint or chamomile. Put a teaspoon of dried herbs in a teapot and pour a cup of boiling water over them. Then place the cover on the pot and allow the tea to steep for 10 to 15 minutes. Herbalists refer to herbal teas as infusions. You can also brew tea from a fresh herb such as mint. In this case, use two to three teaspoons of herb per cup. Steep for 10 to 15 minutes. Pour yourself a cup of tea and sit back and relax while your brew gently takes effect. Brewed teas keep for up to 2 days in the refrigerator.

•If you're working with a specialist in traditional Chinese medicine for your menopausal symptoms, you may be given packets of various plant materials that need to be cooked to extract their

healing compounds. Such preparation is called a decoction. The herbs are boiled in water for as long as 20 or 30 minutes. The plant material is then strained out, leaving the medicinal liquid. Roots, barks, and seeds, which are challenging, are usually prepared in this way, as they require more prolonged exposure to heat to extract their active compounds.
•You may decide to take herbs in the form of prepared *tinctures*. H erbs are kept for about two weeks in a solution of alcohol and water, both of which act as solvents and dissolve nearly all the relevant ingredients in the plant. The herbs are then removed, and the remaining liquid is the tincture. Because a mixture is a liquid, herbs in this form are more easily absorbed. However, medicines sometimes have a bitter taste.

You'll find many herbal medicines sold in *tablet* and *capsule* form. This is the most convenient way of taking herbs. However, some women who are already supplementing with various vitamins and minerals decide that they do not want another pill to swallow and prefer the liquid tinctures and ex- tracts. Herbs often work best in combination. Various hormone-balancing and menopause formulas can be found in health food stores, shops specializing in spices, and mail orders. A good recipe for menopausal women might contain such herbs as alfalfa, black cohosh, red clover, chaste berry, false unicorn, ginseng, holy thistle, liquorice root, sarsaparilla, and squaw vine.

Using Herbs Safely

The medicinal herbs commonly taken today have been used for treating ailments for hundreds if not thousands of years. The poisonous herbs have long been removed from the herbal pharmacy. In addition, over the centuries, the best ways to take herbs were carefully recorded, as well as any side effects. However, whenever you take herbs, you still need to use caution. Some herbs are dangerous if you have certain medical conditions, take particular drugs, or are pregnant or nursing. Work with a skilled professional, such as an herbalist or naturopathic physician.

Even if you self-prescribe, be sure to check with a specialist who can assess the herbs you plan to take. In addition, do not exceed recommended dosages. The labels of many herbal products give recommended amounts. These are generally safe to follow. If you have any questions about dosage, consult with a trained specialist.

Watching for Side Effects

When taken appropriately, herbs should not cause significant side effects. If side effects do occur, they are usually relatively benign and may include nausea, diarrhoea, and skin reactions. However, an individual may experience more severe side effects such as hypertension and allergic reaction. Before taking any herbal preparation, you must know the signs of toxicity and watch for these. If you are taking any form of drug or medication, be sure to inform your supervising physician that you plan to take herbs so that a potential drug-herb interaction can be avoided.

Chapter 9: Living a fulfilled life through menopause

Physical activity feels good because it is good for you! Movement benefits the body, the mind, and the spirit. Children instinctively know this and relish being physically active. Un- fortunately, many adults seem to have forgotten the pure pleasure of moving their bodies. Exercise benefits female health in several ways. Physical movement increases the circulation of the blood, allowing more nutrients to reach target tissues and cells. Exercise stretches stiff tendons and makes them more supple. Physical activity causes more oxygen to reach the brain, stimulating mental function. A good workout dispels stress, a known trigger for menopausal symptoms, and exercise can help maintain an average weight. Being overweight in itself can lead to hormone imbalances and related menopausal problems. It is no wonder many women are finding that regular exercise can help reduce symptoms of menopause and that exercise needs to be a component of an overall plan of self-care. Hot flashes, irritability, sleeplessness, fatigue, and memory can all be improved with physical activity. In addition, exercise can help lower the risk of degenerative diseases, including osteoporosis and heart disease, which women are more prone to as they age.

Ancient and Modern Forms of Exercise

Certain types of exercise are particularly effective in keeping women well. Some involve slow movement, controlled breathing, and even meditative thought. These include yoga, tai chi, and qigong (pronounced "Chee Kung"). These disciplines, all three originating in Eastern cultures, developed over centuries and consisted of various postures and choreographed movements that target specific anatomy components. Certain poses, in particular, nourish female health. These practices can leave you feeling wonderfully vitalized after a single session. However, a consistent use over many months brings even more significant benefits, healing the body and building a foundation for good health. But women at midlife also need active, vigorous physical activity that can stimulate the system and support the healthy functioning of organs, tissues, and cells. Jogging, aerobics, and weight-bearing exercise are prime examples of the modern and Westernized approach to exercise. These can help temper signs of menopause and also exercise the heart and strengthen bones. Sometimes the walk from the sofa to the front door is the most challenging exercise of all. Make up your mind to give yourself the gift of exercise. Remember how good it can feel to stretch your legs and draw in the fresh air if you want inspiration. Remember the exhilaration you feel after exercising, how clear your mind is, and free of worries. Take a walk right now!

Getting Started

You may be thinking that you hate jogging, and you'll never be caught in an aerobics class with a bunch of 20-somethings. But don't let this stop you from exercising altogether. If you don't already exercise, the first step is simply to begin, and it doesn't matter how. Start with a walk through the mall. If you want company, you may even be able to join a mall-walking group. These are cropping up in cities subject to exceptionally cold or hot weather. Residents require indoor exercise space away from the elements. Member's window-shop and chat while exercising! Tackle a creative home project that you've wanted to do, perhaps some landscaping. Or buy a gallon of paint and give a wall in your home a new lease on life. Such projects will have you moving muscles you didn't know were there. Live out a fantasy. Take that tap dancing class you've always thought about. If you can't keep your feet from moving while watching a Fred Astaire movie, per- haps ballroom dancing is for you. Have you always wanted an adventure vacation rather than sitting at the beach? Contact environmentalist groups or ask around at your local science museum or university for opportunities to do some fieldwork as a volunteer. Tagging turtles, sifting through sand, or cleaning up the environment in some way can get you moving! The following sections take a closer look at specific types of exercise suitable for women and maybe just what you need.

Yoga for Women

Yoga is an ancient practice, developed in India thousands of years ago, and yoga continues today to be a powerful and effective way of maintaining health. Take advantage of yogic wisdom to facilitate your passage through perimenopause and into menopause. Yoga is a form of exercise, a meditative discipline, and a means of becoming at peace with yourself. As Robert Birnberg, a yoga instructor based in Los Angeles, explains, "Menopause can be confronting to women who see this as a sign that their youth is over and that they are no longer of use in the society. But yoga offers women a way to accept and be comfortable with the changes menopause brings and experience menopause from a new perspective. Yoga postures and breathing techniques can help a woman establish a healthy relationship with herself. And yoga draws a person's attention inward, rather than to outside problems, which with time, can feel less of a burden." The physical moves of yoga consist of two parts: disciplined breathing and postures. These poses are held for a given length of time, measured in breaths. You can perform yoga at virtually any age because yoga offers various exercises and routines tailored to any level of physical ability. Even women in wheelchairs do yoga.

Yogic Breathing

A primary focus of yoga is to enhance the benefits of breathing, taking in oxygen, which will bring life to the cells, and the expelling of carbon dioxide. This toxin must be removed from the body. If you are like most people, your breathing is shallow. Your body barely moves as you inhale and exhale. Yogic breathing is deep and full. On an inhale, the chest expands. On an exhale, the abdomen pulls in, moving the air out through the lungs. There is research that following a regular pattern of breathing can control hot flashes. In a 1992 study published in the *American Journal of Obstetrics and Gynaecology,* researchers experimented with paced breathing to reduce hot flashes. Thir- ty-three women who were experiencing frequent hot flashes were asked to slow their breathing. By doing so, they were able to reduce the frequency of hot flashes significantly. The researchers suggested that such an approach to managing hot flashes could be beneficial for women who cannot tolerate hormone re- placement therapy. Try the following if you feel a hot moment coming on. Slow your breathing and take only five or six breaths a minute, about one every 10 seconds. You may want to practice doing this in advance, counting slowly from 1 to 5 for each inhalation and from 1 to 5 for each exhalation. As you slow down your breathing, you may be able to stop your hot flash in mid-course. Rhythmic, deep breathing also calms the mind and soothes emotions. The mood swings and irritability that may occur during perimenopause can be tempered by modulated breathing.

Yoga Postures for Menopause

Yoga postures evolved as a way of facilitating and enhancing this way of breathing. A pose may involve opening the arms wide and pressing them back. This opens the chest. The following move might be a bend from the waist, which automatically compresses the abdomen and physically initiates an exhale. Yoga poses stimulate circulation, massage and tone the organs and inner muscles, and keep the body limber—a proven way to ensure youthful ageing. It's not hard to find yoga teachers in their 60s and 70s. Some women begin taking yoga classes in their 80s. Practicing yoga also helps balance the endocrine system and evening out the glandular and hormonal changes at menopause.

What about twisting your body into pretzel shapes? This is the mental picture most people have in their minds when they think of yoga. These advanced postures are for the experts, but you don't need to do these to benefit from yoga. Trying to do overly challenging poses can get in your way. In the world of yoga, the struggle is not associated with success, and the motto is not "just do it!" The yoga exercises that will help most with menopausal symptoms are those that you can do while keeping your breathing full and steady, without straining to the point of feeling pain. Some of the most beneficial yoga postures for menopause are described here. As you read through these, you may want to try some of the suggested positions, but resist the temptation. To make sure you don't put too much strain on a muscle or twist your back, take the time first to find a yoga teacher who can show you how to perform these moves safely. Ideally, have a private lesson and work out a series of postures selected from the ones in this chapter suited to your ability and needs. Start with a few simple ones that you can commit to performing regularly, and add more difficult poses only after the first ones begin to seem easy.

INVERSIONS

Yoga postures that involve inverting the body have long been valued for their cooling effect and are known to reduce hot flashes. They also quiet brain activity. If you want to begin with a straight posture, lie on your back with your buttocks close to a wall and your legs raised and resting on the wall. Stay in this position for 5 or 10 minutes, taking long, even breaths and keeping your eyes closed. Next, you may want to try the Supported Half Shoulder-stand (Viparita Karani) and the Full Shoulder-stand (Sarvangasana). However, to reduce the risk of injuring yourself, you need to first experiment with these poses with the help of a yoga teacher. Headstands and handstands are the most advanced of the inversion postures. These positions affect blood flow to every organ in the body, including the endocrine system's glands. Certain places tend to normalize the function of these glands, helping prevent hormone fluctuations, which can trigger hot flashes. When the body is inverted, the venous blood, which is more relaxed, drains out of the legs and into the pelvic area and abdomen, helping to prevent the body from heating up. An inverted posture also helps lower elevated blood pressure and reduces fluid retention, which can occur during perimenopause. This comes about as the pose sends the body a signal that blood pressure has increased. In response, the body quickly takes steps to reduce blood pressure. Blood vessels relax, and excess fluids and salt, which can increase blood pressure, are excreted.

Yoga is also thought to affect the life force within the body, known as *prana*. Inverting the body is said to draw the life force inward, toward the organs, and away from the skin where heating occurs during a hot flash.

FORWARD BENDS

Forward bends are incredibly soothing and calming both to the nervous system and the mind. These movements gently stretch the

spine, promote relaxation, and reduce mood swings and anxiety.
Examples include the Head to Knee Pose (Janu Sirsasana) and the
Standing Forward Bend Pose (Uttanasana). Yoga
teachers sometimes recommend these poses to clear up a case of
the blues. Forward bends are also a symbolic way of expressing
acceptance of the natural changes occurring. A forward bend
places gentle pressure on the abdominal area, including the uterus
and ovaries, and squeezes the blood from these tissues. When you
raise your body and come out of the pose, freshly oxygenated
blood bathes these organs and enhances their function.

TWISTS

After menopause, your body begins to produce a significant
amount of estrogen via the adrenals. The kidneys also become
involved. Yoga poses that require twisting are perfect for
stimulating these organs. Examples include the Half Fish Pose,
which can be done on the floor or sitting in a chair. The idea is to
twist the torso so that you are looking over your shoulder. This
twist involves more than just the spine and comes from deep
within the body. Another type of pose that stimulates the adrenals
and kidneys but takes more agility than an elemental twist is the
Bow Pose (Dhanurasana), which looks like its name. You begin by
lying on your belly, bending your knees, and reaching for your
ankles, which you then grip with your hands and hold for 5 to 10
breaths. These positions stimulate the functioning of the kidneys
and adrenals, including the production of estrogen.

WEIGHT-BEARING POSES

Poses that put extra force on your legs and arms help strengthen
your bones. The Half Dog Pose and the Downward-Facing Dog
Pose (Adho Mukha Svanasana) achieve this. The Half Dog can be
done by placing the palms of the hands against the wall, fingers
leading upward at chest height. You then step back until your
torso is parallel to the floor and your legs are at right angles to the

floor. Your body, the wall, and the bottom together form a square.
In the Full Dog Pose, you bend over with buttocks raised and form
a triangle with the base. Weight-bearing yogic exercises draw
minerals to the bones and stimulate bones to thicken. Yoga also
builds muscle and enhances a sense of balance, which can help
prevent falls and related bone fractures.

ACTIVELY RELAXING

Relaxing muscles can relieve aches and pains, reduce fatigue, and
improve the quality of sleep. This posture is guaranteed to relax
you. Lie on your back, a pose known appropriately as the Corpse
Pose (Savasana). Close your eyes. Relax your neck muscles and
look for any other tension throughout your body. Sink into
the earth. Quiet your breathing and your thoughts and remain this
way for 10 minutes. Just focus on the ebb and flow of your breath.
When you are finished, roll your body to one side and slowly sit
up. This posture is performed at the end of every yoga practice. It
works independently as a substitute for a quick nap. Giving
yourself this downtime strengthens and soothes the sympathetic
nervous system, which helps you to manage stress. Becoming
peaceful is also known to reduce high blood pressure.

SUBTLE MOVEMENTS

This yoga pose (Aswini Mudra) works the vaginal muscles and the
sphincter muscles of the anus. It is similar to the well-known Kegel
exercise. Aswini Mudra helps prevent incontinence and the need to
urinate more frequently, which can begin to develop at menopause.
This pose also helps prevent vaginal infection and dryness. Sit tall,
in a comfortable position, with the spine lengthened. Contract
the vaginal and sphincter muscles as if you are trying to keep from
urinating. Hold this pose for a few breaths, and then relax the pose
for a few breaths. Repeat 5 to 10 times, extending the length of
each contract and relaxation as you become more comfortable with

the carriage. This pose increases blood flow to the pelvic area and tones pelvic muscles in the pelvic floor area.

Chapter 10: Natural and Therapeutic remedies to menopause

For many women, the treatment of choice for menopause symptoms and the pre- prevention of diseases of ageing is hormone replacement therapy (HRT). Most likely, if you discuss menopause with your physician, you will be offered some form of supplemental hormones. However, while many benefits of taking hormone replacement therapy are well known, questions remain about its long-term safety and side effects. As future research provides more information about the pros and cons of taking hormones, physicians may recommend HRT with more certainty. But no matter how much evidence or research a doctor gathers, each woman ultimately must make this vitally important decision for herself, either by discussing the option of hormones with an open-minded physician or, if given a prescription, deciding on her own whether to fill it! This chapter tells you about the various forms of hormone treatment available. It explores the benefits and side effects of these and updates you on current research.

The Beginnings of Hormone Replacement Therapy In 1938, an inexpensive form of estrogen was distilled from plant sources. Prescribed to treat menopause, the hormone could be taken orally and did not require an injection. However, it was not until the 1950s and early 1960s that Robert Wil- son, a physician, popularized estrogen replacement therapy (ERT). With seemingly unlimited enthusiasm, he recommended prescribing estrogen well before menopause began so that a woman would never experience symptoms of the change. He even recommended estrogen for such conditions as acne and "sexual underdevelopment" and often prescribed large dosages. Then in the mid-1970s, case histories began to appear in medical journals showing an association between taking estrogen alone, without progesterone, and an increased risk of developing endometrial cancer. These observations spurred researchers to find a safer way to administer estrogen. Eventually, they discovered that taking progesterone along with estrogen could significantly eliminate this cancer risk. By the end of the decade, hormone replacement therapy was once again given the green light. Today, the most commonly prescribed estrogen, Premarin, is a conjugated equine estrogen derived from pregnant mares' urine. Many women find this method of production an insurmountable obstacle to taking the drug because of the possible mistreatment of the animals. There are also synthetic and semisynthetic estrogen compounds available, including Ogen and Estrace. (For more information on supplemental estrogen, see page 159.)

Benefits of Estrogen and Progesterone

Supplemental hormones offer many benefits, substantiated by a growing body of research. Hormone replacement therapy impacts the reproductive system and can ease and even eliminate symptoms of menopause.

Estrogen

Estrogen can dramatically reduce the frequency and severity of hot flashes after a few weeks of use. ERT also helps a woman avoid the fatigue that may result from persistent hot flashes, as well as night sweats. Moods even out. And supplemental estrogen counteracts the thinning and dryness of vaginal tissue, which can make intercourse uncomfortable. The vagina once again becomes lubricated. A woman's outer skin also becomes moistened and better retains elasticity. Studies show that supplemental estrogen helps restore verbal memory. Initial studies recently completed also indicate that estrogen can lower the risk of developing Alzheimer's and other forms of dementia. Urinary tract infections tend to increase after menopause due to tissue changes. Burning and irritation during urination are more likely. Estrogen can reverse these symptoms. However, there is no proof that estrogen alleviates urinary incontinence, which is common post-menopause. This problem is more related to age than hormone deficiency. Using supplemental estrogen is also one way to reduce the risk of osteoporosis and, in some cases, heart disease. (More information about this is given later in the chapter.)

Progesterone

Progesterone can help reduce hot flashes and, in certain circumstances, is the preferred hormone of choice. When a woman begins to experience her first hot flashes during perimenopause, her estrogen levels may be relatively high, and taking more estrogen would only create more hormone imbalance. Supplementing with progesterone can also prevent excessive menstrual bleeding (menorrhagia), which can sometimes occur during perimenopause if a woman has become anovulatory (no longer producing eggs) or has a defective luteal phase of her menstrual cycle (when progesterone is usually created). However, also be aware that menorrhagia may not be related to progesterone levels. Heavy bleeding can occur for various reasons, including stress, obesity, uterine fibroids, and hypothyroidism.

Using Hormone Replacement Therapy

Both estrogen and progesterone come in a variety of forms. Working with your physician, you can experiment with these to find what works best for you. Here's what you have to choose from.

Supplementing with Estrogen

You have your choice of synthetic estrogens and natural estrogens. There is frequently some confusion about what these two terms mean. For the record, both types of estrogen are synthesized in laboratories. Most synthetic estrogens are made from the urine of pregnant mares. They have a molecular structure that slightly differs from your body's estrogen; thus, pharmaceutical companies can patent these compounds. Natural estrogens, in contrast, have the same hormone configuration as the estrogen women usually produce—that is estradiol, estrone, and estriol.

Types of Supplemental Estrogen and Their Routes of Delivery

You can take estrogen in various forms, whether you are taking estrogen alone or a combination of estrogen and progesterone. The pill form is the most common, followed by the patch and vaginal cream. Estrogens are also available in gels, as sublingual, and as injectable pellets. Premarin, which comes in pill form, is the most frequently prescribed estrogen. This preparation consists mainly of mixed

estrogens derived from a pregnant mare's urine; hence the trade name.   Some
of the hormones, such as *equilin*, are not naturally present in huma ns.   Still,   once ingested,   the   body   converts   these   to estradiol. Premarin was first introduced in 1941 and has been used in many experiments focusing on supplemental hormones.

PILLS

All drugs are taken orally, including estradiol in pill form, move from the intestines, and travel immediately to the liver in high concentration before continuing to other areas of the body. In estradiol, the liver breaks down some of the estradiol to estrone and other forms of estrogen. There can be problems with this route of delivery. Estrogen, once ingested, can accumulate in the digestive tract. Here it can be hormonally transformed by bacteria, which can change the type and potency of the estrogen the body eventually receives. This route of delivery requires that the liver be optimally functioning, which may not be the case. Liver function may not be up to par if a woman's diet is high in sugar, fat, or alcohol and lacks B-complex vitamins. In addition, the pill form of estradiol may not be appropriate if a woman has a history of liver disease, gallbladder disease, clotting problems, or hypertension. The most common form of estrogen, estradiol, can also stimulate the liver to produce large quantities of potentially harmful substances, such as cholesterol and proteins that promote clotting. Because of these problems, purified estrone is sometimes prescribed instead. Estrone pills consist of the compound estropipate, which is available in a generic form, Ortho-Est tablets, and is sold under the trade name Ogen. This product has less of an effect on the liver's production of proteins than other oral estrogens. Premarin is a conjugated estrogen, that is, a mix of types of estrogen. When you take Premarin, you benefit from taking an extensively studied medication. The benefits and side effects are well known. Premarin is also available in a broader range of dosages than any other estrogen product, allowing a physician more options in tailoring a prescription to your needs. Another option is Estratab, an esterified estrone type of estrogen synthesized from soy and wild yam. Estratab has the same potency and uses and is available in the exact dosages as Premarin. Esterified estrogens break down more slowly in the bloodstream, thereby providing a steadier supply of hormones. The usual recommended dosage for estrogen is 0.625 milligrams; however, there are exceptions. For relief of symptoms, some women need as much as 0.9 to 1.25 milligrams of estrogen. To avoid side effects, other women need to cut their dosage to as low as 0.3 milligrams. In the standard protocol, oral estrogen is taken for 25 days each month, followed by a week of no estrogen, before this cycle is repeated. Unfortunately, the break-in treatment can bring on menopausal symptoms such as hot flashes. Another oral

estrogen protocol is to take the pill continuously without a week off. Taking estrogen without progesterone can increase a woman's risk of uterine cancer and is only recommended if your uterus has been removed.

THE PATCH

An alternative to the pill is the patch, a small, round piece of adhesive several inches thick. Each patch holds estrogen that passes across a membrane and is absorbed trans-dermally (through the skin) and into the bloodstream. (The skin is the largest organ of elimination in the body and is also a ready avenue of absorption.) The advantage of the patch over the pill is that the estrogen it delivers is absorbed directly into the general circulation rather than first travel to the liver. Lower dosages can be prescribed. The patch also has a steadier flow of hormones than the pill, more closely mimicking the body's production of estrogen.

Consequently, transdermal estrogen is less likely to trigger menopausal symptoms. In addition, this form of estrogen offers some protection against osteoporosis and heart disease. However, the latter benefit is now controversial. Transdermal estrogen is marketed under the names Estraderm and Climara, which contain estradiol. It is a good choice for women who have had a history of gallbladder or liver disease and high blood pressure and blood clotting unless clotting factors are abnormal. The patch is available in a range of dosages from 0.0375 to 0.1 milligram. The patch is applied directly to the skin on certain critical areas of the body that readily absorb the hormone—the abdomen, the thighs, and the buttocks. The patch must be changed twice a week, and with each application, the patch must be placed in a new location. It can cause skin irritation, but rotating its placement can help prevent this. As with the pill, the patch needs to be used in conjunction with progesterone to reduce the risk of uterine cancer.

ESTROGEN VAGINAL CREAM

Estrogen vaginal cream is applied to the vagina and the urethral area and is thereby absorbed into the bloodstream. Like the patch, this delivery method also avoids the intestinal tract and the liver and eliminates related side effects. While estrogen vaginal cream can affect various parts of the body, it is primarily used to reduce thinning of the vaginal walls and restore these tissues to a healthier and more youthful condition. The cream can increase vaginal lubrication, making sexual activity more comfortable. However, a drawback of vaginal cream is that its effects are not as predictable as other forms of supplemental estrogen. Estrogens can be absorbed into the system in widely varying amounts, determined by the thickness of the vaginal wall. The effect of vaginal cream is also insufficient to reduce the risk of heart disease or osteoporosis significantly. Using a cream can be messy, and the cream may soil

clothing. You could also choose to use a natural estrogen cream, which can be used vaginally and applied to various body areas. The estrogen is massaged into the thin, soft skin of the chest, stomach, inner arms and thighs, and neck. This cream is made from soybeans that contain estrogenic compounds. Natural estrogen cream contains sitosterol, a form of estrone. It offers the advantages of any natural hormone product, and like any transdermal product, it is effective at lower doses. One of the most common estrogen vaginal cream products is Premarin cream. It is applied using an applicator that can deliver 1.25 to 2.5 milligrams of estrogen to the tissues of the vagina; however, smaller doses are often sufficient. Some women benefit most by using estrogen cream every day for a week or two until their vaginal tissue begins to respond. At this point, using the cream only twice or three times a week is usually sufficient. Estropipate, which metabolizes to estrone, is also available as a cream. Suppose you decide to use natural estrogen cream. In that case, the starting dosage is ¼ teaspoon a day, which supplies approximately 1.85 milligrams of estrogen. This dosage can be slowly increased until symptoms abate. You can then reduce the dosage to the minimum needed to prevent symptoms. As with the other forms of supplemental estrogen, you also need to take progesterone to prevent cancer of the uterus. Supplementing with progesterone, at least every three months, can help achieve a balance of hormones and prevent the lining of the uterus from thickening or becoming precancerous.